Acclaim

Responsive Feeding

"Every so often you come across a book that inspires a *yes, yes, yes* response. *Responsive Feeding* is one of those rare gems! From learning to respond to your baby's signals to dispelling feeding myths to proactively addressing feeding challenges, *Responsive Feeding* provides all the tools, techniques, and tenderness parents need to make mealtimes joyful instead of stressful."
—**Lindsey Biel, OTR/L,** coauthor of *Raising a Sensory Smart Child*

"*Responsive Feeding* is a comforting, engaging must-read for all parents, caregivers, and professionals in the pediatric feeding space. Melanie Potock uses her decades of experience and expertise as a feeding therapist to unite the often conflicting camps of baby-led weaning and puree enthusiasts by educating readers about the beautiful simplicity of what is perhaps the most underappreciated concept in pediatric feeding."
—**Malina Malkani, MS, RDN, CDN,** author of
Simple & Safe Baby-Led Weaning

"Melanie brings wonderful insights with her responsive feeding approach, which recognizes the relationship that underpins all interactions, especially feeding, from birth on. This book is a parent-friendly guide, balanced by essential information for therapists. As a feeding and swallowing specialist for infants in the NICU (Neonatal Intensive Care Unit), I am confident that Melanie's guidance and strategies will provide a positive way forward for infants and children with feeding challenges, and those who care for them."
—**Catherine S. Shaker, MS, CCC-SLP, BCS-S,** pediatric
speech-language pathologist

"As moms to five children combined, we can confidently say this book is a must for parents! Melanie brilliantly points out that you have thousands of opportunities to enrich your child's associations to a variety of foods, while simultaneously building lifelong language skills—and guides you in taking advantage of every mealtime. *Responsive Feeding* eases your stress and allows you to reclaim the joy of feeding. Melanie, thank you for this amazing resource for the parent community!"
—Brooke Dwyer, CCC-SLP, and Bridget Hillsberg, CCC-SLP, Speech Sisters

"*Responsive Feeding* is a practical road map to the daunting task that all parents must tackle: introducing a baby to the exciting, sometimes overwhelming, world of solids. Potock's expert guidance cuts through all the myths and anxiety, leaving parents with a true understanding of how to help their children build a healthy relationship with food."
—Larissa O' Loughlin, RN, IBCLC, The Mama Coach

"*Responsive Feeding* is an essential resource for all parents on their feeding journey. Melanie empowers parents to really understand their children's needs and cues, providing loving, expert guidance and instruction to help baby thrive."
—Alex Caspero, MA, RD, and Whitney English, MA, RD, founders of Plant-Based Juniors

"Melanie has masterfully dovetailed the developmental milestones of learning to eat with a parent's more powerful strategy: attaching and connecting through responsive feeding. This book is a must-have for parents who want to start feeding on the right foot and raise children who artfully regulate their own appetite and eating."
—Jill Castle, MS, RDN, author, and founder of The Nourished Child

"*Responsive Feeding* is an absolute gem that will help parents achieve successful mealtimes. As an early intervention provider, I always turn to Coach Mel for feeding-related questions. Now, thanks to this book, I have immediate access to all her expertise right on my bookshelf!"
—Cari Ebert, MS, CCC-SLP, speech-language pathologist and early intervention specialist

"With her decades of experience, Melanie Potock has written the bible on how to safely introduce foods to infants with responsive or infant-led feeding. A practical and easy-to-follow book, Responsive Feeding outlines when, why, and how to introduce foods to your child while reading their cues and readiness."
—**Holly E. Knotowicz, MS, CCC-SLP,** speech-language pathologist and feeding specialist

"I'm beyond grateful to Melanie for providing a new perspective on feeding—being more responsive to your little one's cues. This book includes many feeding strategies that have been helpful in my own feeding sessions. If you're a parent, SLP, or OT, you'll definitely find this book useful for your child and clients!"
—**Grace Bernales, MS, CCC-SLP,** pediatric speech-language pathologist

"Melanie Potock has done it again! This is one of the best books on the market for responsive feeding: It guides you through each phase of development from six to thirty-six months, answers all your questions, and solves feeding challenges. This is a must-read, must-give book!"
—**Erin Geddes, MS, CCC-SLP,** certified orofacial myologist

"Guided by the evidence-based information in *Responsive Feeding*, caregivers can feed their children with confidence. The information for navigating feeding disorders and difficulties while providing a responsive approach is critical!"
—**Autumn R. Henning, MS, CCC-SLP, COM, IBCLC,** founder of Chrysalis Orofacial

"This book will help you create successful and stress-free experiences when feeding your child—especially in the first three years of life—and makes it easy to transition your baby to solid foods! As a mother and pediatric feeding specialist, I wish I had this book when my children were infants."
—**Hallie Bulkin, MA, CCC-SLP, COM**

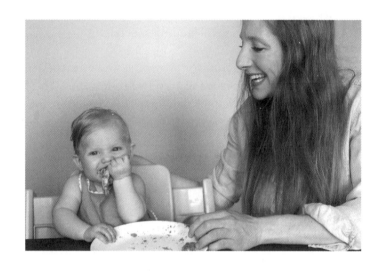

Also by Melanie Potock

Adventures in Veggieland:
Help Your Kids Learn to Love Vegetables

Raising a Healthy, Happy Eater
(coauthor with Nimali Fernando)

Responsive Feeding

The Baby-First Guide to Stress-Free Weaning, Healthy Eating, and Mealtime Bonding

Melanie Potock, MA, CCC-SLP

Foreword by Mitchell H. Katz, MD

THE EXPERIMENT

NEW YORK

The Experiment, LLC
220 East 23rd Street, Suite 600, New York, NY 10010-4658
theexperimentpublishing.com

Library of Congress Cataloging-in-Publication Data

Names: Potock, Melanie, author.
Title: Responsive feeding : the baby-first guide to stress-free weaning, healthy eating, and mealtime bonding / Melanie Potock, MA, CCC-SLP ; [foreword by] Mitchell Katz, MD.
Description: New York : The Experiment, [2022]
Identifiers: LCCN 2021038232 (print) | LCCN 2021038233 (ebook) | ISBN 9781615198368 (paperback) | ISBN 9781615198375 (ebook)
Subjects: LCSH: Infants--Nutrition. | Infants--Weaning. | Baby foods.
Classification: LCC RJ216 .P663 2022 (print) | LCC RJ216 (ebook) | DDC 649/.33--dc23
LC record available at https://lccn.loc.gov/2021038232
LC ebook record available at https://lccn.loc.gov/2021038233

ISBN 978-1-61519-836-8
Ebook ISBN 978-1-61519-837-5

Cover design by Beth Bugler | Text design by Sarah Schneider
Cover photographs by istock.com/chinaview and dreamstime.com/ivanlonan
Author photograph by Carly Potock

Manufactured in the United States of America

First printing January 2022
10 9 8 7 6 5 4 3 2 1

Contents

Foreword by Mitchell H. Katz, MD 1

Introduction 3

Chapter One Ready for Solids the Responsive Way 7
AT 6 MONTHS

This Is Responsive Feeding 16

Understanding Your Baby's Reflexes 24

Understanding the Difference: Gagging versus Choking 29

Pay Attention to Baby's Eight Senses 37

Understanding the Difference: Hunger versus Appetite 44

Get in the Groove with Solid Foods 48

Common Concerns 60

Feeding Myths 62

Chapter Two Building Momentum & Communication Skills 65
6 TO 12 MONTHS

How Babies Communicate 65

One Family, One Meal: Safe Foods to Offer 72

The Right Tools in Little Hands: Utensils, Cups & Plates   82

Pacifiers: Yay or Nay?   93

Common Early Challenges & How to Navigate Them   96

Chapter Three It's the Pace, Not the Race   103
12 TO 18 MONTHS

You Provide, Your Child Decides   106

Simple and Safe Shifts in Nutrition   112

Transitions in Appetite   119

Common Responsive Feeding Scenarios & Types of Eaters   129

Tricky Transitions: Breast, Bottles & More   134

Chapter Four Rounding the Bend   141
18 TO 24 MONTHS

Building More Skill & Ability for Self-Feeding   145

Feeding & Communication Myths   157

Chapter Five Coasting through Challenges   161
24 TO 36 MONTHS

The Natural Fear of New Foods   167

Sugar & Artificial Sweeteners: Restrict or Regulate?   170

The Research Supporting Family Mealtimes   175

Chapter Six Eating Away from Home
& Navigating Family Influences   179

Responding to Strong Opinions from the People You Love   180

Infusing the Flavors of Your Heritage   182

Day Care & Preschool   184

Restaurants   188

Feeding Myths that Impact Development   189

Chapter Seven Red Flags & Special Needs   193

Pausing to Chat with Your Pediatrician   194

Feeding a Medically Complex Child in a Responsive Way   198

Conclusion   211

Acknowledgments   213

Appendix: Resources & Recommended Products   215

Notes   217

Image Credits   229

Index   231

About the Author   244

To the women in my life who paused during their climb to extend a helping hand.

To my husband, who makes every day the best day.

To my children, who keep me laughing and bring me so much joy.

My heart is full because of you.

Foreword

BY MITCHELL H. KATZ, MD

In the first five years, a child is fed approximately ten thousand times. This is daunting to imagine, especially considering that feeding a child is so tied to our concept of being a loving and nurturing parent. At the start we must acknowledge that there are three things we cannot control with a child: We cannot make them sleep, poop, or eat. Yet we invest so much of our identity as a successful parent in what our child eats and how they grow. Their needs are ever-changing as they develop.

At every point along the developmental timeline, a parent must communicate with their child, first and foremost. When babies are born, they are helpless and totally dependent on caretakers to satisfy their basic needs—and that's where responsive feeding first comes in. While we take for granted the complexity involved in getting food from the dish to the mouth to the stomach, understanding your child's abilities will help you, as a parent, present an age-appropriate diet to your child. As a child matures, skills develop that allow them to try more types and textures, and they acquire the ability to self-feed. Responsive Feeding allows you to track their development and gives you the knowledge and understanding to set proper expectations when it comes to food.

As children do not come with an attached instruction manual, it is left to you to learn the stages of your child's development and how to meet those needs. Unfortunately, today, parents are left to map out how they care for their child with search engines and social media, which carry the risk of misleading or incorrect information. We need a source of information that is rooted in experience and fact-based science. In this book, *Responsive Feeding: The Baby-First Guide to Stress-Free Weaning, Healthy Eating, and Mealtime Bonding*, Melanie Potock provides a stepwise, evidence-based reference that will help you understand the developmental stages of your child and guide you in providing age-appropriate, complete nutrition.

With practical suggestions for all aspects of feeding, this book offers ideas from selecting and preparing food to developing proper feeding strategies by managing language—focusing on communication between you and your child—to setting behavioral expectations tied to your child's age and ability. Not only does this book clearly and comprehensively teach you how to feed your child, it teaches communication strategies that begin the day your baby starts solids. It dispels commonly held myths that may lead you astray and emphasizes the importance of bonding during mealtimes.

Enjoy the journey as you join your child in exploring the world of food. With *Responsive Feeding*, together you can share the taste and joy of eating.

MITCHELL H. KATZ, MD, is the medical director of pediatric gastroenterology and nutrition at Children's Hospital of Orange County, UC Irvine School of Medicine.

Introduction

Congratulations! You have a new baby! Your baby's first year of life is an incredible time of growth and development that can often feel like a roller coaster, especially if you're a busy parent. When my own daughters were born, I was elated and overwhelmed all at the same time. In the early months, your child is expected to reach developmental milestones outlined in baby books and parenting blogs and shared by your pediatrician during frequent well-child visits. You'll likely have long checklists to keep track of in the middle of daily routines. It is especially difficult when things aren't coasting along as planned and you feel like you're headed for a bumpy ride filled with uncertainty. Proper nutrition is what helps to lay the strong foundation to meet developmental milestones. Unfortunately, it has become more and more overwhelming to obtain straightforward advice and research-backed information about how to feed your baby in a way that is safe and that promotes their independence and cognitive and motor development.

Know that you are not alone. Parents all over the world have shared similar concerns, and that's what prompted me to write this book for you. Although nutrition is important, feeding your child involves more than a balanced meal. With responsive feeding, you will be able to tune in to vital aspects of human communication and feel confident in your responsibility for feeding your child. Knowing how to read your baby's communication cues and your toddler's often very strong preferences (hello, two-year-olds!) is the key to being a responsive feeder. As a certified speech-language pathologist who has specialized in pediatric feeding for over twenty years, it's my hope that I can help parents uncover the secret to a joyful mealtime: communication.

You may be wondering: What's so different about responsive feeding? Responsive feeding provides opportunities for children to practice independence with less restriction on the parents or caregivers, allowing you to help your child as needed. Gone are the rules to "skip purees" and "only let baby feed themself" that can feel rigid to many families. Responsive feeding allows you to respect their autonomy and decision making on how much they'd like to eat, yet provide assistance based on developmental needs and communication cues. Want to spoon-feed? You can do that with responsive feeding. How about boosting along self-feeding skills? You can do that, too. Responsive feeding is flexible because the focus is on the reciprocal back-and-forth communication that every parent experiences with their child. Responsive feeding has been recognized by the leading children's health organizations for its crucial role in child development and nutrition. Through reciprocal and responsive interactions, it helps improve cognitive and language development in young children.[1]

Think of responsive feeding as a dance. Have you ever been arm in arm with a dance partner, both of you enjoying the music and the movement? Feeding your baby is similar. It's about engaging your baby, anticipating their moves, and taking turns to lead the choreography. You respond to baby's communication, and baby responds to yours. Because you are in tune and present in the moment, you will connect and flow, making for a beautiful experience! I am here to guide you from starting solids to heading off to preschool with a brand-new lunch box. Feeding trends come and go, but babies don't change the way they communicate.

This book is designed to answer the most common questions about feeding babies and toddlers up to age three. I'll be debunking myths while offering practical tips on making mealtimes joyful and less stressful. I will teach you a no-nonsense, straightforward approach to responsive feeding that's focused on nurturing, trust, and communication between you and your child. My mission is to provide you with the knowledge and confidence to share the love and traditions that food can bring to the entire family. In the first six months of life, you've created a bond with your baby while feeding breast milk or formula. Responsive feeding with solids enhances that bond and builds trust between you and your little one using a flexible, research-backed model proven to raise mindful, healthy eaters.

Chapter One

Ready for Solids the Responsive Way

· AT 6 MONTHS ·

You have just met with your child's pediatrician for the six-month well-child visit. Your baby is meeting their developmental milestones with ease, and you receive the green light to start solid foods. How exciting it is to see your baby sitting up by themself and finally showing interest in what you are eating! But as you're leaving the doctor's office, you realize that after being caught up in the emotion of baby's latest milestone, you forgot to ask: What foods should you start with? What time of day is best to offer a meal? And how much should your baby even be expected to eat? So many questions are left unanswered in your mind, and feelings of anxiety start to creep in. Don't worry! We're about to learn everything there is to know about starting solids.

In the past, it was recommended that babies start solids as early as 4 months, but modern guidelines from the American Academy of Pediatrics (AAP) and the World Health Organization (WHO) state that breast milk, if possible, is the ideal source of nutrition for baby for about six months.[1] If you are unable to give your baby breast milk, formula is the ideal substitution to help your baby thrive. Offering exclusively breast milk or formula until 6 months allows your baby to get enough vitamins and minerals for body and brain growth. However, baby's iron stores begin to deplete between 4 and 6 months in breastfed babies, and the AAP recommends an iron supplement starting at 4 months.[2]

Starting solids too soon might affect your baby's gut health and cause an imbalance of important nutrients for growth. By 6 months of age, the healthier and more mature gastrointestinal system will be ready for a variety of foods, and therefore better able to absorb nutrients. Shortly after, your pediatrician may feel there will be no need for iron supplementation. In this chapter, you'll learn when to start offering solids and how to recognize the crucial windows of opportunity. You will learn to watch for signs of readiness and all about the flexibility of responsive feeding. Following a model that is both parent-responsive and baby-led feels so good!

When should you start offering solids? Of the many factors to consider, your baby's immune system, sensory system, and motor development are just a few.

The immunity window

Baby's immune system plays a key role in the best timing for first solids. It's challenging to find the perfect window of opportunity when reading various studies on the topic, but it appears to be as baby approaches 6 months of age. Scientist Alice Callahan, PhD, summarizes several studies beautifully as follows:[3]

> When a baby begins eating solid foods for the first time, new proteins bombard [their] gut. There seems to be an optimal window—a sweet spot—for the immune system to learn about these proteins. Introduced too early, and it appears that the gut and immune system are not yet equipped to respond appropriately. But introduce too late, and the window may have closed; the immune system might only be able to react to the

protein, instead of learning to tolerate it. Introducing gluten to a baby before 3 months of age or after 6 to 7 months seems to increase the risk of celiac disease.[4] Similarly, introduction to cereals, both rice and gluten-containing grains, before 4 months or after 6 to 7 months has been associated with a greater risk of type 1 diabetes."[5]

Your baby's gut health has been shown to play a crucial role in overall health and the development of diseases.[6] The immunity window is one piece to consider and may be of special importance if your family has a history of celiac disease, type 1 diabetes, or other factors that may increase the risk for these diseases, such as Down syndrome. The sweet spot may be just before your baby turns 6 months of age.

The flavor window

There is a sensitive window of time when babies are more likely to accept new tastes and more complex flavors. Research indicates that this magical flavor window is between 4 and 6 months.[7] Given that it's best to wait till about 6 months of age for optimal gut health and motor readiness for solids (as you'll see in the next section), the flavor window is slowly beginning to shut the moment first solids are introduced! However, with repeated exposures as your child grows, they will become an adventurous eater.

The key is to start early, offer a wide variety of flavors and textures, and don't stop offering if baby doesn't seem to like a particular food. Most parents offer foods three to five times, decide their child doesn't like it, and completely stop offering it.[8] "What's the point?" they often ask me. "He won't eat it." The point is that eventually your child will take a taste if you parent consistently. Offer small portions of less-preferred foods beside the more desired foods. Provide about a teaspoon for kids to sample or simply to have on their plate and explore as much as they'd like, throughout their childhood. Repeated exposures to new tastes start from baby's first bites but continue into adulthood.

The motor window

Mother Nature has a timeline for your baby's motor development. Waiting too long to introduce solids or not offering a variety of safe textures can hinder baby's ability to learn how to bite, chew, and swallow safely. This motor window of opportunity aligns with the integration or fading of baby's oral motor reflexes, discussed later in this chapter. Babies make the most progress learning to bite, chew, and swallow from ages 6 to 10 months. It's certainly not perfected until age three, but kids make huge strides in progress during this motor window.[9] In a 2017 randomized control trial, eight-month-old babies who were exposed to diverse, safe textures (including purees and mashed foods) for four weeks significantly improved their ability to chew a piece of soft carrot or potato for the first time. There were no changes in their ability to manage new mashed foods, presumably because those foods were already mastered in the age-appropriate timeline of 6 to 7 months. In short, babies need to be exposed to textures, ideally during the optimal motor window, to learn to manage them safely.[10] In a large study of 9,360 babies, researchers discovered that babies introduced to lumpy solids at 10 months or later developed feeding delays. By 15 months, they were "significantly less likely to be having family foods when compared to those introduced between six and nine months."[11]

Feeding is a developmental process. We don't keep infants in strollers or other baby carriers all day long, because it would hinder gross-motor development, like learning to crawl. That's only common sense. The same is true for waiting to introduce solids. The parent's responsibility is to open the classroom in a timely manner and provide safe and age-appropriate opportunities to learn about food. Most typically developing babies are ready at 6 months old. Some will take to the lessons immediately, and others will be content to explore and consume little at first. But without the exposure, many kids will develop a feeding delay.

Signs of Readiness

One of the most crucial factors to consider when starting solids is your baby's level of readiness based on gross- and fine-motor development. It all starts with your baby's core muscles. Because baby's tummy and back muscles are so much stronger than just two months ago at the previous well-child check, you'll notice that your baby's head is steadier on their shoulders and they can sit on their own with minimal support. Babies might not have teeth yet, but they enjoy bringing safe toys to their mouth while seated upright. This overall trunk stability is what your baby needs to operate the fine motor movements of biting, chewing, and swallowing. Bringing toys, and eventually food, up to the mouth independently are fine-motor movements. Gross-motor stability in the trunk is essential for babies to create accurate fine-motor movements and to reach across the center of their body ("crossing midline") to grab bits of food scattered in front of them. Watch for the following signs and share your baby's progress with your pediatrician to determine if they are ready to start solids:

Necessary signs

- Head and neck control
- Trunk stability
- Sitting up with minimal support
- Crossing midline
- Bringing toys and fists to mouth

Other positive signs, but not always indicative of readiness

- Showing general interest in food and others' eating
- Lip smacking and open mouth in anticipation
- Reaching for caregiver's food
- Doubling their birth weight

When motor skills are considered, most typically developing babies are ready for first solids at about 6 months of age. For optimal nutrition in the coming months, it's best not to miss this crucial time to help baby explore a variety of tastes, textures, and subtle changes in temperature. In fact, waiting past the age of 9 months indicates a delay in feeding development. This is partially due to every child's need to learn from reflexive movements. From 6 to 12 months, babies learn to eat by reflexes that move the lips, tongue, and other muscles in the mouth. These reflexes teach baby to move their tongue to the left and right with food in their mouth, propel the food backward, and more. Those same reflexes integrate (seem to disappear) into the nervous system over time, and unless baby has experienced attempting to eat with the support of those reflexes, they must figure it out on their own. In other words, baby needs to have safe food options in their mouth in order to experience the oral muscles responding to various reflexes—and to learn to do it purposely on their own. We'll go into more detailed information on the exact reflexes that teach baby specific feeding skills later in this chapter.

Myth Busting: Baby is ready for solids when the tongue-thrust reflex has disappeared.

This common myth is seen on popular feeding websites and across social media. The tongue-thrust reflex, which is closely related to the infant suckling reflex, causes the tongue to move forward and back to express milk from the breast. That movement shifts *slowly* starting at about 6 months of age and morphs into an up and down movement at the end of the first year. The tip of the tongue eventually finds the spot on the roof of the mouth (where you make the "d" sound), pressing *there* instead of pushing *out* to swallow. The reflex gradually disappears between 6 and 12 months as baby gains more control over the reflex, because they are being exposed to different textures of food.

Responsive Feeding Your Way

There are a variety of feeding styles and methods to introduce solids to your baby. Deciding which method to pursue can feel overwhelming, and parents often tell me they feel trapped when they start one style and it isn't going as smoothly as expected. They report that they feel judged by friends and family if they don't choose a traditional method that family members are familiar with or more modern methods that are popular on social media. Because I am a speech-language pathologist, I am a firm believer in communication being the key to any relationship, especially the feeding relationship. No matter what feeding style you choose, you can learn the fine art of communicative, responsive feeding. And yes, it's fine to do a hybrid feeding approach or to shift from a style that isn't working for you! In pediatric feeding therapy, where I work with children with special needs, one of the first items I share with parents is a printed treatment plan—but it is only a plan. Your baby will let you know if you need to tweak your feeding plan, because you will be listening and responding to baby's cues. This is true for any child, with any level of feeding skill. In any school, kids learn differently, but if the teacher is a top-notch communicator who is flexible in their teaching methods, the kids learn to love school. Think of mealtimes like food school, where we bring joy and connection to the classroom while learning about new foods.

Most pediatric feeding therapists categorize feeding styles into three distinct methods: The first method, typically referred to as "the traditional approach," was likely popular with your parents. This involves beginning with ultrasmooth pureed textures and progressing to chunkier purees over the first few months of starting solids. Pieces of soft foods are introduced after the hierarchy of smooth to chunky purees is established. The second method, referred to as "Baby-Led Weaning" (BLW), is a model first introduced by Gill Rapley and Tracey Murkett. In contrast to starting with purees, this method emphasizes skipping purees and introducing from the very start most solid foods that the rest of the family is enjoying. In addition, BLW stresses the importance of allowing baby complete independence in the feeding process. In my clinical experience, I've discovered that most parents want to engage in a third method or hybrid approach.

Whatever method you choose, the key to developing a healthy relationship with food is to learn to read your baby's cues and communication style, and then respond mindfully. Rather than following one specific method, let's focus on the most common questions and concerns that you may have and provide safe solutions based on the most crucial aspect of parenting: communication between parent and child. That is the foundation for responsive feeding.

How I Came to Responsive Feeding

In the early '90s, I experienced a pivotal moment in my career that eventually would lead to writing several books on pediatric feeding. Today, that moment shines brightly in my mind as I write this latest book for you. A position for a speech-language pathologist (SLP) became available in my city's hospital within the Neonatal Intensive Care Unit (NICU). The role of the SLP was to partner with an occupational therapist, physical therapist, physicians, and other NICU staff to help premature and/or medically fragile infants grow and thrive. As part of the NICU team, my primary job was to teach parents how to read the frail baby's cues and respond in a supportive manner, whether it be during feeding, while introducing infant massage, or during their child's first bath. However, the overarching and looming goal was for the physician to discharge the tiny patients based on their ability to breast or bottle feed, or, sometimes, return home with tube feedings as the baby continued to learn how to coordinate sucking, swallowing, and breathing. The babies needed to eat without experiencing stress and expending so much energy that they would lose weight. Unfortunately, despite my efforts, the parents often felt pressure from other professionals or family members (and sadly, insurance companies) to get their baby to eat so that they could bring their baby home. When parents focus on *getting* children to eat rather than their *learning* to eat, whether it's a premature baby or a fussy toddler, it may work in the short term. But it will quickly backfire, causing the child to associate eating with negative experiences and to develop negative memories that influence future mealtimes.

Drawing from the work of international experts, including Catherine Shaker, MS, CCC-SLP, BCS-S, Erin Sundseth Ross, PhD, CCC-SLP, and Joy V. Browne, PhD, I taught parents and other professionals who cared for the babies the concepts behind cue-based feeding and developmentally supportive care. Like responsive feeding methods, these two models of feeding infants emphasize the importance of "reading the feeding," a phase first coined by Shaker.[12] In the American Speech-Language-Hearing Association's (ASHA) article titled "Reading the Feeding," Shaker explains: "Cue-based feeding assumes that preemies actively communicate through their behavior, which provides information to the caregiver about the infant's thresholds of stress versus stability. The caregiver, in effect, partners with the infant during feeding: The infant offers behavioral and physiologic signs to a caregiver, who interprets them, selects contingent interventions that support and strengthen the infant's efforts, and respects the infant's limits."[13]

In contrast, volume-driven feeding is where the pressure to get baby home is driven by the urgency to have the baby ingest a specific volume. Developmentally supportive care and cue-based feeding allow babies to communicate exactly what they are capable of at each feeding attempt. Furthermore, "In volume-driven feeding, success is measured by how much an infant ingests, and caregivers may use strategies intended to empty the bottle without regard to what the infant communicates. . . . Volume-driven caregiving tends to feed past the infant's 'stop' signs, which say, 'I want to stop, I am done.' Failure to respond to the infant's communication may lead to maladaptive feeding behaviors, learned feeding refusals and long-term feeding aversions. Caregivers often pass on this volume-driven philosophy to parents, for whom feeding becomes something they do 'to' their infant, instead of a relationship-based experience through which communicative interactions build trust."[14]

What I learned in my early years as a pediatric feeding specialist in the NICU is that feeding is, first and foremost, based on a nurturing, loving, and responsive relationship. I've never forgotten that. At its best, it is a reciprocal experience, a dance where each partner contributes to the flow and the rhythm. The key to an infant's or child's relationship with food is a positive relationship with their feeding partner. How do we develop that essential partnership, where both the parent and the child enjoy mealtimes together and volume consumed is not the ultimate goal, yet the child will grow and thrive? The answer is simple—by nurturing our children and adopting a flexible approach to feeding, known as responsive feeding.

This Is Responsive Feeding

If you pay close attention, you'll find that your baby has many ways of communicating with you, even though they cannot talk yet. Though it can be confusing at first to try and decode these signals, with time and patience you'll begin to discover your baby's unique cues. When you're able to respond to them in a calm and nurturing way, a greater bond and connection can be made between you and your child, especially at mealtimes. This is responsive feeding at work and is a smaller piece of the bigger theoretical model that is responsive parenting.[15]

Researchers Maureen M. Black of the University of Maryland School of Medicine and Frances Aboud of McGill University describe the similarities of responsive parenting and responsive feeding in this way:

> The development of healthy eating behaviors depends on both healthy food and responsive parenting behaviors. With origins from anthropology, psychology, and nutrition, responsive parenting reflects reciprocity between child and caregiver, conceptualized as a 4-step mutually responsive process:
> 1) the caregiver creates a routine, structure, expectations,

and emotional context that promote interaction; 2) the child responds and signals to the caregiver; 3) the caregiver responds promptly in a manner that is emotionally supportive, contingent, and developmentally appropriate; and 4) the child experiences predictable responses.[16]

Using Black and Aboud's multistep process, here's how this might work:

1. A loving routine is established in a predictable environment (your child's mealtime).

2. Your child communicates hunger (e.g., gesturing for food via sign language or reaching toward others' food; fussing after a reasonable period of not eating).

3. You respond quickly and calmly (setting up in the high chair for a meal of solids).

4. Your child experiences predictable, positive responses from you, reinforcing their attempts at communication.

Sounds simple, right? In theory, it is. It just takes consistent practice to get the feel of the back-and-forth communication that makes it such a delightful experience! Like learning to dance, the first few steps may feel awkward and require a lot of concentration to make sure they're in the right sequence, but soon, everyone is dancing in sync and having a lovely time.

Both Baby-Led and Parent-Responsive

As the name implies, feeding responsively requires that you react to your baby's cues and signals. This could be before a mealtime even starts, or between bites. Responsive feeding does not—and should not—mean that you are in complete control of a meal but instead, that you are responding to support your little student as needed. Though your baby is making the first move in the dance that is a mealtime, you remain engaged, supportive, and connected throughout the process. Caroline Weeks, an RD at the Mayo Clinic, shared her thoughts on this form of mindful feeding, calling it "meditation at mealtimes." You must be present, listening, and watching for your baby's attempts to communicate their wants and needs, and respond accordingly. In some instances, your baby will start the conversation, in other cases you might initiate it. In all cases, however, the communication is mindful and built on trust.

Helping Children Thrive

Many children around the world are faced with food insecurity and nutrition concerns such as growth issues, underweight and overweight, and/or inadequate intake of certain food groups or vitamins. In the most recent Dietary Guidelines published by the US Department of Health in 2020, it was found that zinc, potassium, and choline were underconsumed by older infants and that 77 percent of infants fed human milk had inadequate iron intake.[17] Maintaining responsive feeding patterns can promote more developmentally appropriate growth and weight gain. A study including over 90 pairs of mothers and their children ages 12 to 17 months concluded that use of responsive techniques such as positive verbal encouragement made children over twice as likely to accept bites of a meal.[18] Keep in mind that the child always makes the decision whether to accept a bite, but in the case of responsive feeding, mothers are responding to their baby's cues with positive verbal encouragement, rather than using words to bait the child into taking a bite. It's a subtle difference that we'll continue to explore throughout this book.

Responsive Feeding Is Flexible!

As a professional feeding therapist, I've noticed that part of parents' confusion between traditional feeding and BLW may lie in a key disagreement between the two models when offering purees. In using the traditional feeding method, purees are viewed as an essential step in feeding development. In some BLW circles, purees appear to be viewed as a detriment to a baby's development.

As a clinician, my role is to educate parents on the pros and cons of various feeding strategies. I believe that purees have a purpose. Although it's not necessary to introduce purees first, there are some benefits that can be helpful to a child's development. Your baby has been practicing suckling from the breast or bottle for several months, and we can build on that skill by offering a slightly thicker liquid like smooth, pureed, and flavorful vegetables. According to Shaker, an international expert and specialist in infant swallowing, "purees help intrinsic tongue muscles develop, preparing babies to learn to chew and swallow more efficiently."[19] Are purees essential to develop safe swallowing skills? Not necessarily, but they don't hinder feeding development, as long as we also offer other developmentally appropriate foods and can support feeding skills at the same time. Lastly, purees can offer an element of convenience and can be prepared in a way that allows for greater nutrient density per bite. That's the beauty of blending a variety of foods and flavors!

Hesitant to offer purees? It may be that you're hesitant to hold the spoon and present it to baby because you want to follow BLW practices. The issue may not be the puree, it might be the method of delivery—and it's OK to feel that way! Flexibility is key in responsive feeding. Try offering safe solids dipped in purees, such as a full-size, thick carrot for baby to suck and explore. If your child is already showing signs of being able to bite through crunchy foods, omit the large carrot and offer a softer, steamed narrow stick (about the size of your pinky finger) dipped in yogurt or hummus. Little fingers are a fun way to learn about purees, too, because baby gets dual sensory feedback from the nerves in the hands to the nerves in the mouth. There's nothing like dipping fingers into a mild guacamole to develop a future love of avocado toast! Learn more about the world of purees and the different ways of offering them to baby in the next section.

Responsive Feeding with Purees

Have you ever seen a caregiver attempt to "airplane" a spoon of purees into a baby's mouth and try multiple relaunches when the baby turns their head with pursed lips? What about when a spoon is used to wipe away a messy mouth between bites and the baby resists the frequent and often uncomfortable cleanup? These are two examples in which responsive feeding with purees is ignored. It's not the puree. It's the lack of reciprocal communication that's the issue.

The airplane game is not a terrible game if the players are both eager to play. When baby turns their head or purses lips, they are communicating no. Responsive feeding respects baby's internal cues and the resulting body language. Wiping a messy mouth might appear helpful, and if baby doesn't appear to be uncomfortable, it's probably fine. Still, I avoid it.

Think about what that feels like: Would you like a spoon scraped across your lip or chin after every bite? Instead, try a gentle but firm pat with a damp washcloth on occasion, which most babies prefer, rather than scraping. Plus, the experience of food around the mouth is not dysregulating unless a child has sensory processing difficulties. And, in that unique case, a therapist works specifically on helping a child learn to tolerate that sensation, as it's an appropriate part of this developmental stage for kids this age. Messy is helpful, as we will discuss in the section on the eight senses (page 37). But as a parent, I understand that messy isn't always practical. Watch for the upcoming section on whether bibs are a good idea (page 50).

There are many ways to offer purees, based on responsive feeding techniques:

Present a "loaded spoon" to baby. Scoop puree onto a pre-spoon and hand it to baby to self-feed. Another option is to place the spoon on the table or feeding tray for baby to grasp when interested.

Let baby use their fingers. Purees have an added benefit when it comes to early feeding skills. Babies who are ready to start solid foods can bring their own hands to their mouth to explore fingers, thumbs, fists, and palms. Spreading a bit of puree on the high chair tray or a clean tabletop for our babies allows them to explore the texture, subtle temperature changes, and other aspects of tactile input with both their hands and mouth at once. The dual sensory experience provides more input to the nerves in the hands and mouth, providing more data to the brain. The more information that baby can file under "positive food experiences" in the brain, the more information they can compare and contrast with new food experiences. By watching baby reach for and explore the purees and responding via your own participation and modeling (e.g., you dab your finger and lick it) you're inviting baby to continue to explore purees and bring the purees to the mouth. Feeding is developmental and requires multiple steps for baby to learn to be an adventurous eater. Responsive feeding includes inviting the baby to participate in the lesson but also in being willing to wait for baby *to be ready* to be a participant.

Allow baby to come to you. When you are spoon feeding, hold the spoon as if it were floating in the air. Allow your baby to initiate the bite. Lean slightly forward with a look of expectation, instead of directing the spoon into the mouth simply because that little mouth was open. Remember to smile and use eye contact to keep baby engaged in the dance. It's easy to get distracted when the world is so new and exciting! Learning to decipher the difference between distraction and lack of hunger comes naturally if you're willing to wait with the spoon in the air, giving baby time to respond at their own pace. Hunger will drive that pace, and as baby's appetite subsides, you'll see less interest in the spoon.

In chapter two, I'll discuss proper spoon-feeding techniques in more detail (page 83). It's important to not scrape food onto the roof the baby's mouth, which is a common mistake.

Responsive Feeding with Handheld Solids & Mashes

Like purees, soft handheld solids such as a slice of ripe avocado or a well-steamed, soft carrot stick can be presented in a responsive manner, whether you're following a baby self-feeding approach like BLW or more traditional feeding methods.

Watch, listen, and observe your baby's attempts at communication. No matter how you present food options, the key is to respond to your baby's body language and vocalizations. Consider the following examples:

Scenario #1: Baby is seated in the feeding chair, alert and ready to explore food. The parent might choose to offer strips of baked sweet potato and a few pea-size cubes of moist, soft mozzarella for baby to rake up and attempt to put in their mouth. If baby drops the food during the learning process but does not appear distressed, the parent responds by waiting, gently remarking "Oops!" and letting baby take the lead and try again. If baby repeatedly drops the food and appears frustrated or abandons the task, the parent may opt to coat the strips or cubes in cracker crumbs (see box) and offer again.

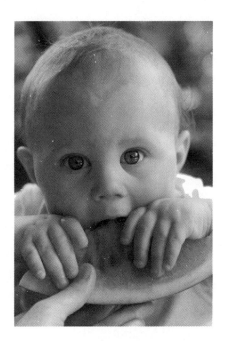

Whether offering baby a loaded spoon or a safely-cut slice of watermelon, as you hold the fruit still, watch for baby to lean forward, sometimes grasping the food for stability, and bring it to their mouth. Baby is telling you, "I'm ready to explore that!"

<u>Scenario #2:</u> Baby is seated in the feeding chair, alert and ready to explore food. The parent might dip a textured pre-spoon or beginner utensil in smashed avocado and hold it patiently in front of baby to grasp or lean forward to mouth while the parent continues to hold the utensil. The parent waits and watches for baby to indicate that they are ready to accept what is presented. That visual cue, the loaded utensil, might also be accompanied by a smile or a verbal cue: "Yummm . . . avocado!" But it's always baby's decision whether to continue the interaction.

<u>Scenario #3:</u> Baby is seated in the feeding chair, alert and ready to explore food. The parent holds two spoons, both pre-loaded with two different mashes, and waits for baby to pick one to grasp and mouth. When baby stops exploring the spoon with their mouth and lets it go, the parent picks it back up, loads it again with food from the tray, and offers the two options again. This is the time to be mindful of baby's ability to use both hands and cross midline (cross the left hand past the chest to the right side, and vice versa). Alternate the

two spoons occasionally so that each mash is presented equally on the left and right to ensure that baby is not dependent on any food offered to one side. Reading baby's cues also helps with fine and gross motor development!

Understanding Your Baby's Reflexes

Feeding is a developmental process. It's just like learning to crawl, then walk, then run. There is a specific timeline for feeding milestones, which is dependent upon reflexive movements—that is, teaching babies to suck, bite, chew, and more. When babies have difficulty with feeding development, it may indicate a feeding delay or disorder. (See chapter seven to learn more about red flags for feeding delays and feeding disorders, page 196.) Many of the reflexes are present at birth and then slowly integrate into the nervous system in the first and second years of life. These reflexes are essential to help baby grow and thrive via breast and bottle feeding, and later contribute to learning to eat solids. It's important to understand how several of the reflexes that are present from birth support your child on their journey to healthy eating.

Why are reflexes so crucial in feeding development? Reflexes teach baby the motor movements, and then baby learns to perform each movement with intention, on their own. At first, the reflexes are obvious, though they appear to fade as baby's volitional movement takes over. Volitional movement is learned movement that we do on purpose. For example, when your doctor gently taps your knee with a rubber hammer, your lower leg jumps. That's reflexive. But when you intentionally raise your lower leg, that's volitional.

There are seven reflexes at play when baby learns to eat solids.

Rooting Reflex

Feeding: You may remember this reflex during the first month of baby's life, when it is most active. When babies are first learning to breast or bottle feed, this reflex helps them find milk. Touch baby's lips or cheeks with the nipple and baby's head will turn and move toward the stimulation! The mouth opens reflexively, ready to accept the nipple. After that first month, baby will begin to turn toward the breast or bottle and open their mouth intentionally. The reflex fully integrates between 3 and 6 months of age.

Communication: The rooting reflex helps to build muscles needed for baby to turn their head toward your voice and to build stability in the jaw and facial musculature for talking.

Suckling Reflex

Feeding: The suckling reflex is the cutest! Watch your baby's tongue move rhythmically under a nipple. That movement is a reflex called a suckle, and soon it will emerge into a true sucking pattern that becomes intentional. You'll notice a forward-backward tongue movement when baby is suckling at the breast or bottle. That wavelike tongue movement reflexively extracts liquids and then propels the food down the throat in a rhythmic, predictable fashion. The same movement is used to suck on a pacifier or fingers. At about 3 months of age, suckling begins to morph into a true sucking pattern. It's a more advanced tongue movement, in which the front of the tongue moves independently from the rest of the tongue. When baby is sucking, the cheeks and lips are engaged in order to propel more advanced foods as baby begins solids, and to move larger volumes of liquids needed for baby to grow. If you see your six-month-old sucking smashed sweet potato off their fingers, that's usually intentional and not reflexive. They learned to do that because of the early suckling reflex. You may still see occasional reflexive sucking during breast or bottle feedings, but after 6 months of age, the majority of the time sucking is done with the purpose of self-soothing or eating.

Communication: The tongue is composed of eight muscles—four extrinsic and four intrinsic. The extrinsic muscles provide stability and attach to bones, while the intrinsic muscles create different shapes to produce vowels and consonants. The suckling and sucking reflexes contribute to more than just feeding skills; as the muscles work together, reflexive movements become coordinated movements that are then combined with voicing. Early reflexes contribute to the process of speech development and are manifested in baby's coos, babbling, and first words.

Tongue Reflex

Feeding: Sometimes referred to as the tongue-protrusion reflex, this is the reflex that helps keep a young baby's airway safe. It pushes food or objects out of the mouth. At about 4 months of age (coinciding with the gradual emergence of the sucking reflex), the tongue reflex begins to fade away very slowly. But it can take up to six more months and may occasionally be seen after the first birthday! Baby will begin to use protrusion on their own at about 6 months of age, the same time that you are introducing solid foods. You'll also observe the reflexive protrusion periodically. That makes interpreting these movements a bit tricky! Don't rely on the tongue-protrusion reflex to always protect baby from larger pieces of food that may slide down the throat or get lodged in the airway. Likewise, don't interpret food being pushed out of the mouth as a signal that baby doesn't like the food. This gradual shift from reflexive to volitional movement will come into play as you introduce new textures and shapes of food.

Communication: Toddlers who continue to protrude their tongue tend to develop a forward tongue resting posture that affects speech development. Articulation, or the ability to pronounce words correctly, is a developmental process, just like feeding. The two influence each other because feeding and speech utilize the same muscles and rely on similar movements. Watch for more information on how to ensure that your toddler's tongue movement matures appropriately in chapter three, where I will be discussing bottles, pacifiers, and finger sucking.

Transverse Tongue Reflex

Feeding: "Transverse" simply means that the tongue extends across the midline of the mouth or moves from side to side. Like the tongue protrusion reflex, the transverse tongue reflex helps baby learn to control food in the mouth. The reflex is first seen at birth, when baby's tongue will move toward anything that stimulates the side of the tongue. When your baby is first learning to self-feed with handheld foods, you'll see the tongue moving toward anything placed on the left or right gumline. That reflexive "side swipe" teaches baby how to lateralize the tongue, working specific muscles to eventually place food onto the gums and later onto molars for chewing. Just as important, baby will learn to retrieve that same food after it's chewed and then swallow. If you're spoon feeding, you can help baby learn from the reflex by presenting the food to the gums on the left or right sides, alternating with each bite. Expect volitional movement at about 9 months and mastery by age two.

Communication: Side-to-side movement of the tongue is essential for speech development. Try talking just by moving your tongue forward and back. It's difficult to do and you'll sound like you have a mouth full of marbles! Many children receiving speech therapy require guidance on how to move the tongue in six directions: up, down, forward, backward, and to one side or the other. When kids learn to combine those six directions of movement, making contact in their mouth in the appropriate spots and synchronizing the flow, they can pronounce words clearly.

Swallowing Reflex

Feeding: There are three phases to swallowing: oral, pharyngeal, and esophageal. The oral phase is when the food is being chewed and prepared for swallowing before the tongue gathers it to be swallowed. The pharyngeal phase is when the food enters and travels down the throat. The final phase, known as esophageal transit, simply means the food goes down the esophagus (food pipe), bypassing the larynx (voice box) to enter the stomach. Babies begin swallowing amniotic fluid reflexively while in the womb. Learning to swallow on purpose requires understanding the concept of swallowing, which you can begin to teach at about 18 months of age. Watch for a fun way to teach this concept on page 154. Shortly after baby's first birthday, a mature swallow pattern is established (see page 93). The swallowing reflex never integrates, since we need to swallow saliva throughout the day and night. Humans swallow up to 900 times every 24 hours!

Communication: When children learn to talk, they have to manage their saliva at the same time. Speech pathologists often help young children coordinate the movements needed for speech with the need to swallow during conversations and eliminate drooling.

Biting Reflex

Feeding: Have you noticed that when you place your finger in an infant's mouth, they will bite down and then release over and over? It's like they are gnawing on your finger—luckily they don't have teeth! That reflexive moment is termed the biting reflex for a reason—it's the first step to learning to chew! Baby will gain more control of the reflex between 5 and 9 months when solid foods in a variety of safe textures are introduced. The reflex then integrates between 9 and 12 months. This is why introducing only purees and lingering there can cause a feeding delay. With the reflex gone, baby never gets the chance to practice chewing. Soft cookies or crackers that melt with saliva are an ideal food to activate the reflex and in turn, to learn to bite and chew volitionally.

Communication: Up-and-down jaw movement is essential for speech development. The biting reflex works the muscles that open and close the jaw. The jaw provides the stability for the finer movements of the face, including tongue and lip movements needed to pronounce long strings of syllables in conversations.

Gagging Reflex

Feeding: Thank goodness for the gagging reflex! It acts as a protective mechanism to prevent choking, although it is not foolproof. Fortunately, it never integrates (adults need the gagging reflex, too) but is more easily stimulated in young babies than adults. In infants, the gagging reflex will occur if a nipple is too long or if your baby is highly sensitive to oral input. When babies are ready for solids and are practicing with a variety of safe textures between 6 and 9 months, the gagging reflex has begun to shift and is found on the back third of the tongue. Gagging cannot be done on purpose and is always reflexive. Kids may imitate a gag, but a true gag involves multiple structures—the soft plate rises up, the tongue lowers with force, and the jaw drops forward as the mouth opens. Involuntary muscle contractions in the throat are visible as the larynx rises up.

Communication: Starting from infancy, provide your baby with teethers and chewies that reach to the center of the tongue. Baby will learn to move all the muscles of the mouth thanks to the tongue reflexes mentioned earlier, while desensitizing the overt gag reflex, allowing it to move toward the back of the tongue by age one.

Understanding the Difference: Gagging versus Choking

Gagging and the body language that indicates choking signal caregivers when baby may or may not need help. Understanding the difference is essential to knowing when to intervene.

What is gagging?

Gagging is nature's way of trying to protect your baby's airway. It's important that you know that it's not foolproof, but it is relatively reliable if parents offer safe foods. For babies who are just starting solids, gagging is a natural response to new tastes, new textures, and subtle temperature changes, especially cold temperatures. As noted in the section on reflexes, gagging is a reflexive attempt to push anything forward that is getting too close to the airway. It signals a loss of control of the food, but it does not signal that the airway is blocked. As babies learn to control the food in their mouth, they won't activate the reflex as easily. If baby is getting consistent practice, the gag reflex begins to shift posteriorly, bit by bit, over the next two years.

The most significant difference is typically observed between 6 and 9 months of age, with gags becoming less frequent after the ninth month. This is partly due to baby's gross- and fine-motor maturation, but it's also because baby has been stimulating the tongue and entire oral cavity with fingers, with strips of food, and as they manipulate food in their mouth. This stimulation trains the brain to ignore the tactile input unless the brain senses a loss of control at the back of the throat, just before swallowing. That's why, as adults, we tend to gag on a piece of parsley or foods like a stringy piece of spaghetti that get stuck on the back of our tongue. That's too close to the airway, and the brain takes over to try to expel the intrusive food.

When baby gags, try your best to stay calm. Watch baby carefully, but maintain a gentle, reassuring posture and facial expression. Talk softly to baby, saying simple phrases like "You can cough" or "You can push it out with your tongue." You may see baby's face turn pinker, eyes tear slightly, or sometimes they may spit up a tiny bit, but in general a gag is quickly resolved. You'll be able to hear baby making gagging noises or coughing, an indication that air is moving through the airway and there is no obstruction. Give your child a few seconds to relax, and it is likely they will just resume eating. Most important, do not intervene. Putting your finger in a child's mouth may push the food farther back and elicit true choking. Patting their back may do the same. Wait, watch, and wear a comfortable look. Model calm. Observe for any signs of true choking.

What is choking?

Choking is vastly different from gagging. It has little to no sound because the airway is partially or completely blocked. Here is yet another reason why responsive feeding and consistent mealtime interactions are so important for children. When parents are taught to simply put whatever they are eating in front of the baby and let baby lead, that's oversimplified and dangerous advice. A choking child may be openmouthed, wide-eyed, and drooling, with bluish skin around their lips or eyes. Audible gasps, faint noises, or wheezing may be detected, but there will be a clear look of panic on the child's face. Act quickly, using techniques from your CPR training.

Responding to Gagging and Choking

I've never met a parent who wasn't afraid of their baby choking, myself included when it came to my own daughters! In this book we'll walk through the steps to help you and your baby feel more confident as you start your journey to solid foods. Because you're practicing responsive feeding, which emphasizes reading baby's cues and maintaining communication throughout the meal, you'll be more attuned to your baby's facial expressions, gestures, and body language. Gagging and choking call for two very different types of response based on your interpretation of each scenario.

> TIP: Every parent would benefit from enrolling in an infant CPR course (live or on-demand) to ensure that their baby is safe both in and out of the high chair. Get trained, along with babysitters and older siblings, in CPR and choking first aid, like the Heimlich maneuver. The Red Cross offers a reference guide, public classes in most hospitals, and online courses and instructional videos.

In general, babies tend to gag most often during the first few months of trying solid foods. How much gagging is too much gagging? Observe baby carefully, and if you notice signs of distress or distrust because of the loss of control of food due to gagging, then that's too much. It will vary from child to child, and in my experience babies who gag a few times per meal recover quickly and continue eating, learning to manage the food through positive food experience and as motor skills develop over time. Although not a hard and fast rule, babies who gag frequently may become hesitant eaters with time, as persistent gagging is not a comfortable experience and can lead to gastroesophageal reflux, irritation of the esophagus, and possible vomiting.

Gagging and choking are two quite different events and there are myths and truths associated with both gagging and choking. To help parents and professionals understand the difference and to dispel the myths, I explained it this way in a published article[20]:

Myths

1. **Coughing while eating signals choking.** Typically, occasional coughing while eating means the child had trouble coordinating the swallowing mechanism and is attempting to expel any residue from the airway and surrounding area. To cough, air must be moving through the airway, so a cough is often a good sign of airway protection. However, be on guard for continued coughing or a significant change in breathing pattern during or after the episode.

1. **Gagging on food means my child is choking.** Gagging is a reflex also helpful for protecting the airway. Although we don't want children to experience repeated episodes of gagging or any negative association with food, the occasional gag occurs when the brain detects a loss of control of the food in the mouth. Still, an active gag reflex is not a foolproof safety mechanism. A child's airway is narrow, and food can still become lodged or inhaled much more easily than in an adult.

2. **My baby's "tongue thrust" will protect them from choking.** Babies move their tongues in a forward/backward movement when breast or bottle feeding. When solid foods get introduced, this anterior/posterior movement seems to push food out of baby's mouth until baby learns to propel the food to the back of the mouth for swallowing. Purees help babies learn to manage a safe swallowing pattern, and other soft, handheld foods—avocado or slivers of peeled roasted sweet potato—can gently support feeding skills development. But don't rely on a baby's tendency to push food out before learning to chew and swallow. Learning to eat is a developmental process. Offering foods too advanced for a child's developmental stage increases the likelihood of choking, especially given a young child's unique anatomy.

3. **Raising the hands above the child's head stops the coughing or choking.** Raising arms when someone coughs might make the situation more dangerous. The motion of the arms influences the motion of the child's neck and trunk. In turn, the food causing the coughing can shift and block the airway.

4. **Pat a child's back when they're coughing.** Remember, coughing isn't choking. Patting a child's back when they cough might cause the offending food to fall into the airway and block airflow.

Truths

1. **A person choking often makes little to no sound.** Always stay present and observant while a young child eats. If the airway becomes blocked, little to no air can pass through the vocal folds. Your eyes most likely will see the choking before you hear anything, if at all.

2. **Call 911 and perform lifesaving measures** if a child has trouble breathing, presents with a change of color anywhere about their face or suddenly begins to drool—even if you hear other vocal sounds.

3. **Food can enter the larynx, trachea, and/or lungs for a variety of reasons.** Known as "aspiration" or "silent aspiration," depending on the circumstances, this inhalation of food causes immediate as well as delayed complications. Even if a child isn't choking, aspiration can cause life-threatening issues over time. Bring the following delayed symptoms to the attention of the child's primary health care provider immediately:

- Difficulty managing saliva.
- Wet, "gurgly" voice quality.
- Mucous buildup after eating or chronic congestion.
- Multiple episodes of chronic low-grade fever.
- History of pneumonia or frequent respiratory infections.
- Consistently coughing during or after eating or drinking.
- Fear around eating.
- Decreased interest in eating.
- Weight loss or apparent poor growth.
- Consistent discomfort or irritability just before, during, or after eating or drinking.

Gagging Can Signal What's about to Happen: Choking

Babies can gag and then choke, or they can choke without gagging first. Although gagging is considered "good" by many professionals, too much of a good thing is, frankly, never a good thing. If your child gags frequently and appears uncomfortable, talk to your pediatrician. If your child has just one choking episode, always contact your pediatrician that day to discuss exactly what happened. It's notable for their medical chart, even though it may never happen again. If it happens twice, those specific details may help solve the mystery of why it's happened twice and prevent a third occurrence.

Choking Hazards for Babies & Older Children

The AAP recommends that parents avoid serving these foods unless safely cut for babies and older children up to age four.[21] Preschoolers have very limited attention spans, making it easy to choke, and their esophagus is still quite narrow.

- Whole hot dogs: Instead, cut into strips the width of your pinky finger, then chop into pea-size cubes.

- Nuts and seeds: Instead, chop finely and stir into oatmeal or baked goods.

- Chunks of meat or cheese: Instead, serve soft pasteurized cheeses or grate harder cheeses, being careful to serve just a few strands at a time. Harder cheese easily forms into a ball in the mouth, which can cause choking.

- Whole grapes: Instead, quarter or finely chop (if grapes are very large).

- Hard or sticky candy: Just avoid them and offer softer sweets after age two.

- Popcorn: After age three, kids can have one popped kernel at a time, but who is really going to monitor that? Be especially aware of popcorn in a dark movie theater where the attention is on the film. Remember, choking will most often have no sound.

- Chunks of peanut butter: Instead, spread thinly.

- Chunks of raw vegetables: Instead, soften via roasting, stir-frying, steaming, or blanching well. Try shaving carrots, jicama, or other crunchy raw vegetables with a mandoline to create sheets of veggies for children who have molars.

- Chewing gum: Just don't offer it till after age four. It's an easy one to avoid, since it doesn't show up at meals or snack times. If you're a gum chewer, be consistent in your response to requests to try gum. "Sweetheart, you'll be able to chew gum when you're four. I promise we will have some then!" Introduce gum by tearing a stick in half. Avoid gumballs or large chunks of bubblegum.

Choking Hazards until Baby Has Molars

In addition to the recommendations noted on the previous page till age four, it is crucial that parents be aware of these unique choking hazards till baby has molars. Avoid serving the following foods until after age one and then only if you are feeling comfortable with baby's chewing skills:

- Raw, leafy greens: Instead, soften and chop via roasting or steaming.

- Individual corn kernels: Instead, smash each kernel or serve a cooked and cooled ear of corn. Corn kernels are too fibrous for baby's gums to break down without your help.

- Raw peas: Instead, serve cooked and smashed slightly.

- Large chunks of doughy, soft bread: Instead, toast and cut into strips.

- Fibrous foods like celery, pineapple, or asparagus stalks: Steam or roast to soften and finely dice. The heads of the asparagus are soft enough for littles, but the stalks present a problem unless cut safely.

- Chunks of watermelon: Watermelon can be very challenging for babies because each bite creates added "water" in the mouth. Managing water and the pulp at the same time can cause coughing and sometimes aspiration of the food. Instead, smash the watermelon and serve with a spoon, cut into small pea-size cubes, or let baby gnaw on a thick piece of the rind with a thin portion of pink watermelon flesh attached.

Pay Attention to
Baby's Eight Senses

My colleague Lindsey Biel, OTR/L, coauthor of *Raising a Sensory Smart Child*,[22] taught me to think of a child's sensory system as their own personal GPS, helping them navigate through new experiences. As children grow and learn, we always consider how their eight senses contribute to their willingness to participate in novel experiences. It's vital that parents understand the influence of each sense so that they can respond to baby's reactions to new foods in a supportive and loving manner. Parents are often familiar with the five senses that we teach in school, the senses of sight, sound, smell, hearing, and touch. But there are three other senses that babies utilize to learn about food: the sense of proprioception, the vestibular sense, and interoception.

The sense of sight

You may have heard the phrase "We feast with our eyes," and it is true for young babies, too. In fact, within the first few weeks of birth, infants begin to associate the rooting reflex with the sight of the breast. Reflexes and our sensory system are intimately related. Simply brush the side of your infant's cheek, and baby will reflexively turn toward the stimulation, mouth wide open! Thanks to that reflexive experience, paired with the sense of sight, baby quickly learns that when they spy Mommy's bare breast, it's time to open wide and feast.

As baby matures, they'll continue to use their visual sense in response to food. Babies as young as 3 months of age have learned to recognize familiar objects, and you'll see their faces light up at the sight of a favorite toy! That ability is carried over at 6 months of age, when baby first begins to explore solid foods. Watch your baby reach for favorites on their high chair tray and reach across the table for a food they have learned to love that happens to be on your plate!

With each new opportunity to learn about food, the brain stores or files the experience. By keeping mealtimes joyful from the very start, each sensory experience will be filed under "positive experiences with food," and that's essential to raising an adventurous eater. Humans learn from experience, and we compare memories with new experiences to decide if we will be safe and if it will be pleasurable. The goal is to make sure that baby has so many positive memories around a variety of foods that when they do encounter an unpleasant moment (vomiting, gagging, bitter tastes, and so on) they move on without hesitation, knowing that most food experiences are delicious and fun!

Responsive feeding encompasses all the sensory opportunities that food presents, including vision. Describe what you see as baby reaches for a new food or as they gaze at it with curiosity. To build vocabulary, use single words or short phrases, followed by at least three to four seconds of "pause time" to allow baby to respond. Repeat the same phrases occasionally, to help baby learn from repetition. This method of communication has been shown to boost language development in babies and toddlers. Babies also need to hear typical conversational speech throughout the day, but these shorter descriptions of what you see happening provide context while supporting language skills.

Here's an example of what you might say, see, and hear with smashed blueberries on the high chair tray, using short phrases and pauses to prompt baby to communicate with gestures and vocalizations:

Parent: "Yummm . . . blueberries." (pause)
 Baby reaches for blueberry.
 Parent: "You got it." (pause)
 Baby tries to rake up blueberry into fist.
 Parent: "Yummm . . . blueberries." (pause)
 Baby brings smashed berry up to lips.
 Parent: "Berries on lips!" (pause)
 Baby giggles.

Parent puts a blueberry on own lips: "Berries on lips!" (pause)
Baby pushes the blueberry into their own mouth.
Parent: "Yummm . . . blueberries." (pause)

The sense of touch

New tactile sensations are encountered from the moment baby enters the world. From being swaddled for the first time to being held against a parent's chest with that first skin-to-skin contact, each sensation converts to sensory data stored in the brain. While "touch" is a sensation that involves the largest organ of our body, our skin, we also experience similar tactile input in our mouth and down the throat. Humans have thousands of nerve receptors that detect temperature and texture. From the very first day of life, baby encounters the sensation of warm milk. The types of sensations on our skin and inside the oral cavity and throat are vast. In general terms, tactile input can be described as calming, tickly, or alerting, to name just a few. These descriptors apply to food as well. Warm soup is calming, carbonated water is tickly on the tongue, and biting into a lemon alerts the nervous system!

From the day we start solids to well into adulthood, we use our sense of touch when interacting with new foods. Consider the first time that baby discovers a piece of warm, steamed sweet potato. By squishing it in their palm, smearing it on the table, and pressing it onto their chin with each attempt to get it to their mouth, they discover what it feels like before it hits their tongue. That preview via messy encounters at mealtimes is vital to support baby's willingness to try new foods throughout the toddler years.

Responsive feeding isn't just responding when baby takes a bite but embracing every moment of exploration. Use the same type of short phrases or single words described here to label baby's tactile experience. For example, when presenting the soft sweet potato, the conversation may sound like this (remember to use a tone, pitch, and timbre that is soothing and inviting for baby to participate):

Parent: "Sweet potato . . . warm." (pause)

Baby holds the sweet potato and places it on her lips.
Parent: "Warm kisses." (pause)
Baby giggles and kisses the sweet potato.
Parent: "Momma kiss!" (pause)
Baby giggles and brings potato to Momma's lips.
Parent: "Warm kisses! Your turn!"
Baby kisses sweet potato, and parent pauses, waiting for next cue from baby.

Fingers and hands can do more than touch, they can sign, too! To learn more about signs to use with baby at mealtimes, refer to chapter two (page 68).

The sense of sound

Speech is typically heard via the sense of sound, and language is a rich component of what bounces off the eardrum and is then interpreted by the brain as sound. Your child's brain categorizes all sorts of sounds (not only speech) to help make sense of the world. When feeding responsively, it's your job to respond to both speech and language (body language, too). In fact, some of baby's first words are often the sound that something makes, such as a truck that goes "vroom" or a dog that barks "ruff." Words that represent sounds to the adults ("choo choo") may represent the object (train) to baby. Labeling the sounds or imitating sounds helps baby build language concepts and adds a fun element to feeding time!

Parent drops baked pumpkin cubes onto baby's plate: "Plop!" (pause)
    Baby squishes the pumpkin between their fingers.
    Parent: "Squish!" (pause)
    Baby giggles and squishes another piece.
    Parent: "Squish!" (pause)
    Baby giggles and brings palm up to mouth to lick.
    Parent: "Lick . . . I hear you lick the pumpkin!" (pause) "Lick!"

Keep in mind that for children who are easily overwhelmed by background noise, it may be helpful to take a sound inventory of the feeding environment. Is the ceiling fan whirring above the high-chair or the neighbor's dog barking during lunchtime? The sounds that adults tune out can be the ones that distract young children from the joy of exploring new foods. Just like learning any new skill, auditory distractions can impede the learning process.

It's interesting to note that the sounds that an adult hears while dining influence their perception of taste. Dr. Charles Spence, a leading researcher in this area, studies how the sound a food makes when we bite and chew impacts our desire for more. He also studies how sounds in the background environment (like the sound of crashing waves in a seafood restaurant) influence how we rate the taste of the food at that restaurant. While these adult concepts are years beyond what an infant may find meaningful, there is proof that the sense of sound is a vital component to enjoying the flavor and the overall sensory aspects of mealtimes.

The sense of smell

The olfactory sense is essential for most children to genuinely enjoy food, and there are two ways to detect those pleasant aromas. First, humans get a whiff of a new food as it enters the mouth with the scent entering the nostrils. Second, we get another completely different version of that aroma when it mixes with remnants of other foods, bacteria, and saliva inside the mouth. That secondary aroma travels up the back of the throat to the olfactory center in our brain.

Stuffy noses or medical conditions that impact a child's ability to smell food can affect language acquisition, too. If a child can't smell a flower, how do they know what a "flowery aroma" means? If a child can't smell a mild yet slightly spicy curry, how do they comprehend words like "spicy," if they can't experience the spice? Does it matter if they can taste the mildest spices? Yes, it does. That's where the sense of taste and smell are intimately related.

Modeling how lovely a food smells will help your child understand the concept of aroma, especially if you first tie the concept to taste. Starting at about 8 months, lean over your plate and breathe in deeply through your nose.

Parent: "Mmmmm . . . smells delicious!"
   Baby watches as parent pauses and breathes deep again.
   Parent: "Smells yummy!"
   Baby giggles and tries to sniff.
   Parent: "I'll hold it for you. You can smell it." Parent holds the food
by baby's chin so they can smell it, modeling a deep inhale through
the nose.
   Parent: "Delicious!"

The sense of taste

You may be familiar with the five types of taste that humans can
detect on the tongue: salty, bitter, sweet, sour, and umami. Today,
research suggests the possibility that there may be a sixth recognized taste, known as fatty.[23] However, what's most important isn't
the limited repertoire of tastes, but the endless variations in flavor.
Flavor combines the gustatory sense (taste) and the olfactory sense
(smell). In short, taste plus smell equals flavor. If you can't smell,
you can't experience flavor, but you might be able to experience the
tastes of salty, bitter, sweet, sour, and umami. Those tastes are not
complex enough to maintain an interest in food, but once we regain
our sense of smell, the possibilities are endless when it comes to
flavors!

   How, then, can we respond to babies who are just learning language and still describe so many different flavors? As parents, we
tend to stick to two words when talking about flavor with our kids:
"yucky" and "yummy." Toddlers like these two words, too! But those
are words that describe our reaction to the taste or flavor.

   For babies in their first year, it's best to use simplified vocabulary,
as described on pages 39 and 40. As baby approaches 12 months,
make a conscious effort to begin to use more descriptive words for
flavors, such as "It tastes buttery" or "creamy" or "sour" but always
with a smile on your face. Children interpret the meaning behind

words by watching our facial expressions and listening to the tone of our voice. Although baby won't be using this more advanced vocabulary on their own for quite some time, they'll begin to associate your pleasant expression with the descriptors.

You may remember the five senses noted so far from your grade school days. However, there are three more senses that we pediatric therapists learn about in depth in graduate school. The vestibular sense and the sense of proprioception work in unison to help children know where their bodies are in space and how to grade fine- and gross-motor movements. The sense of interoception is an internal sense that helps kids detect a sensation like hunger.

The vestibular sense

Our sense of balance and movement, originating in the inner ear, is known as the vestibular sense. It is the foundation for all fine-motor skills, and includes biting, chewing, and swallowing. Raking up strips of avocado is a fine-motor skill, as is learning to pinch a tiny pea between the thumb and forefinger before bringing it to the lips. Your child would never be able to do that if their sense of balance was dysregulated. Learn more about how to support your child's emerging fine-motor skills and the vestibular system in the upcoming section on how to position baby in a high chair (page 49).

The sense of proprioception

How does baby know how to bring a slice of ripe cantaloupe up to their mouth when they can't see their own face? How do they know how to connect that little fist of cantaloupe with their lips? It's the magic of proprioception, or a little human's awareness of where their body parts are resting or moving in space. The joints and muscles in our arms, hands, fingers, and jaw send signals to the brain to interpret how much strength, effort, and age-appropriate coordination is required to maneuver that yummy morsel from tray to tongue. The sense of proprioception and the vestibular sense work closely together, helping baby stay balanced and develop coordinated movements to eat all kinds of foods with fingers and utensils.

The sense of interoception

The mysterious sense of interoception is studied in occupational therapy and neurology. In essence, it means that humans can sense internal cues, and learn to respond appropriately. For example, young children can sense when they need to go to the bathroom and eventually no longer need diapers. Infants can sense when they are hungry and cry in a specific way to indicate hunger to their caregivers. Children with special needs and some medical conditions may have difficulty tuning in to these internal cues. When it comes to hunger cues, most typically developing children are quite good at detecting hunger, but appetites vary.

Understanding the Difference: Hunger versus Appetite

Hunger is what you feel. Appetite is your response to that feeling, though it's not always an accurate response to our sense of hunger. I certainly experience that disconnect when I eat way too much at Thanksgiving dinner! Although most babies are born with the ability to detect internal hunger cues and stop eating when satisfied, it is our response to their appetite that is critical in practicing responsive feeding. Responsive feeding supports the child's ability to develop appetite regulation, while allowing for the occasional extra servings at special events (because it's just so delicious!). It's important to acknowledge that sometimes we eat a delicious food just because we love it. No one should ever feel bad about that. But as babies are learning to monitor their own satiety responses, our guidance as parents can make all the difference, even with the more hesitant eater.

In the book *An Appetite for Life*, authors Clare Llewellyn and

Hayley Syrad explain that children may still differ in how they respond to both hunger and food, and may have distinct eating styles that may range from a limited to an avid appetite. This internal drive to eat is shaped by their environment, and that includes your behavior when they eat (or don't eat) what you expected. The authors highlight four crucial components to responsive feeding practices that support the development of "good appetite regulation and a healthy relationship with food" [23]:

1. **Let your child decide how much they want to eat and don't pressure them.** For children with limited appetites who may not be as eager to try new foods or are more hesitant eaters, pressuring can lead to anxiety around food, food aversions, and feeding disorders. For children who are eager eaters, pressuring them to consume more teaches them to ignore their internal hunger cues and satiety signals.

   Examples of unintentional pressuring include requiring that kids finish all the food on their plate, requiring certain foods to be eaten (e.g., vegetables) before getting more of a favorite food, and using phrases like, "It makes Mommy happy when you eat all your green beans."

2. **Don't worry about limiting certain foods.** Your job is to decide what's on the menu. (We will explore this concept more in chapter three, page 106.) Covert restriction means that your child is completely unaware that you're not allowing certain foods, because they simply don't appear on their plate. For example, your six- to twelve-month-old is unaware that you're not allowing them access to honey (because it's toxic to babies and will be introduced when they're older).

   Overt restriction means that the child is very aware of the restriction—and it may backfire because the child develops an even greater desire for the "forbidden fruit." For example, baby can eye the package of crackers on the counter as a parent feeds him and keep reaching and fussing to get their favorite crackers. The parent's overt response is, "We will have crackers after we eat our vegetables," which only sends the message that kids can have the preferred crackers as a reward for eating vegetables.

3. **Offer age-appropriate portion sizes.** If baby indicates that they would like more after enjoying the small sample (about a tablespoon at a time), then offer a bit more.

4. **Offer food in response to hunger and for no other reason.** When we offer food for other reasons, such as comfort, entertainment, or to control behavior, it lays the groundwork for emotional overeating.

Of course, sometimes food appears outside of snack and mealtimes. There are times we eat more than what we need because it's delicious or it feels special. This happens at community events, play dates, and on holidays. But 90 percent of the time, it's best to follow the four responsive feeding guidelines noted above.

Hunger and Satiety Cues

From 7 to 12 months of age, detecting when your baby is hungry may not be so difficult. By now, you've had six months of practice, and have been responding with either the breast or bottle. Now that baby has begun to enjoy solid foods, detecting when they are full and ready to get down from the feeding chair can be more challenging. In fact, a recent study showed that mothers tend to be more responsive to their child's hunger cues than signals that they are full.[24]

Babies this age are easily distracted, have limited attention spans, and may not communicate wants and needs as effectively as even a toddler can. Watch for the following hunger cues to determine if baby wants to eat:

- Eager expression or excitement when they see food
- Leans forward in anticipation, often with an open mouth
- Reaches or points to food
- Attempts to self-feed

- Accepts parents' offerings happily and with ease

Once baby is full, satiety cues include:
- Gradual slowing down in terms of interest and participation
- Turns head or arches body away from food
- Pushes food away or throws food
- No longer opens mouth when food is offered
- Clearly more interested in anything but eating (distracted, playful, fussing)

Why is it so important to be mindful of baby's satiety cues? The AAP states that parents who practice responsive feeding are more likely to raise children who have a healthier relationship with food and healthier bodies because of it. Parents who do not practice responsive feeding teach their children to override their fullness cues and are more likely to have children who are overweight or obese. Children raised in these households may have more difficulty self-regulating their desire for food and may eat for emotional reasons.

How Much Should Baby Be Eating at 6 Months Old?

During the first month of offering solids to your baby, it's tempting to present bites over and over because it's so fun to see baby eating! This first month, however, is more about exploration and learning that there are other foods besides breast milk and formula. During this exciting time, your baby's main source of nutrition will still be those liquid meals. Offer a tablespoon of food at first, watching for baby's signs of fullness or decreasing interest. Then, either offer a bit more or end the meal with a smile and a hug. In the next chapter, I'll discuss portion sizes and the relationship between satiety and calories in each bite.

Get in the Groove with Solid Foods

While there is no hard and fast rule about when to start the first meal, the best time is when your schedule allows for the most consistency and an environment with minimal distractions. Pick a time when you and your baby can genuinely enjoy the experience. Parents often report that mid-morning is a prime window of opportunity.

Breast milk or formula provides most your infant's nutritional needs before the age of one, and so it is important to start with only one or two feeding opportunities per day in the beginning. By 8 to 10 months of age, you'll notice that your baby has gradually transitioned to three solid feedings per day, but this can vary according to baby's appetite and temperament. For more information on balancing breastfeeding and bottle-feeding with your new solid food schedule, see chapter two, page 70.

Remember to trust baby's cues that indicate when they are truly hungry, whether that hunger is directed toward breast milk, the bottle, or newly introduced solid foods. Some of the following common cues may be misinterpreted as hunger: crying, fists closed and brought to the mouth, open mouth, sucking on hands, lip smacking, waking during the night. The dilemma is that these cues *can* indicate hunger. It requires time, practice, and mindful attention to best understand your baby's communicative intent. Trust that you know your baby best. With responsive feeding, there will be trial and error, but before long, you and baby will have established a consistent routine.

Setting the Stage for Happy Mealtimes

The first month of introducing solids lays the foundation for a lifetime of happy mealtimes. Just smile, sit down, and enjoy each other. And remember:

1. Smile and take a deep breath. Your baby will always pick up on your energy, so start by modeling the joy of being together.

2. Set your baby up for success by making sure they are well supported and positioned in the high chair. See the illustration on page 50 to guide you in how to properly position your baby.

3. This is where the dance begins. Every meal from this day forward is a lovely partnership shared by you and your child. Each opportunity may have a different rhythm or tempo; however, the style and approach focus on communication so that you don't step on each other's toes and everyone enjoys the experience!

Think back to some of your earliest interactions with baby. Remember when baby first began to smile with intention? That smile planted the seeds for a lifetime of back-and-forth communication, drawing you in and causing you to smile right back! By the second month of life, baby is smiling and cooing. We, in turn, respond to our infants with each coo and with each smile, and baby expects it. Mealtimes are similar with a responsive feeding model. Focus on offering the food, being present and mindful, and approaching this new adventure with joy! Let your baby take the lead at first. Offer small samplings of safe, squishable options and purees. To learn more and parent proactively, I always encourage reading ahead to help you know what to expect in the coming months. In the next chapter, we'll discuss how babies communicate, signs to watch for that signal yes or no, and other intentional ways that your baby tries to share their feelings with you and, just as important, how to respond.

How to Position Baby in the Feeding Chair

Body language is one of the first forms of communication. When placing baby in the feeding chair for the first time, pause and listen to what that tiny body is trying to say. Baby needs to be upright for safe swallowing, and well supported at the hips and trunk. If baby appears to be steady and upright at first but slowly begins to slump to one side as the meal progresses, that's a sign of fatigue. Babies get tired quickly if they don't have the right support from the start.

In the photo below, see how the baby has an upright back while still allowing for the elbows to rest on the tray? No matter what seat you use for baby, comfort and trunk stability are the priority: 90 degree angle at hips (or pelvis slightly tilted forward), 90 degree angle at knees, 90 degree angle at ankles with feet flat on footrest (smaller babies with shorter legs may not be able to bend their knees yet, but once they can, it's time for a footrest), elbows rest comfortably at tray or table height. I have also noted what features of a chair we find most helpful. For suggested highchairs and feeding seats, please refer to the appendix, page 215.

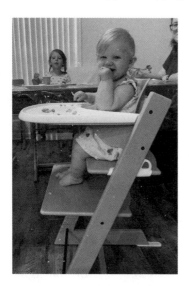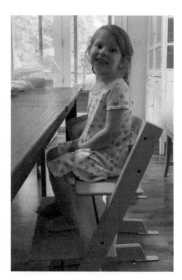

See how big sister, age three, sits in a stable, secure position following the same guidelines as baby? Kids need the right seating at any age!

To Bib or Not to Bib

Feeding specialists prefer that babies not wear bibs and experience the joy of getting messy. Feeling the texture of the various foods with fingers, hands, face, and even that cute bare belly is an important learning experience for your baby's sensory system. When kids can experience food with all the senses, especially touch all over the body, the brain processes and stores that information. It's those sensory files in the brain that lead to eating all kinds of nutritious foods well into the toddler years. Humans use past sensory experiences to compare to new sensory experiences as a means of learning about the world. Offering your baby plenty of opportunities to get messy is always a good thing! But is going without a bib realistic all the time? Of course not. When you need to protect that adorable outfit or just don't have the time for the full-body cleanup, choose a bib that's soft, comfortable, and easy to clean. For ideas, see appendix, page 215. Note that if your high chair comes with straps and buckles, fasten these over the child's bib for optimal safety. When using a full-body bib that won't accommodate buckles over the fabric, make sure you can reach easily underneath to quickly unbuckle baby if needed.

Pre-Spoons and First Spoons

For your six-month-old baby, choose a spoon that baby will be able to grasp with ease and that you can present to baby's mouth if you desire. Look for spoons with short, squat handles for little fists to grasp and that have a flat area for the food to rest yet allow for nice lip closure. That lip closure is vital to help baby learn to manipulate soft foods and propel them back safely to be swallowed. In the next chapter, we'll be exploring all kinds of tools that will support your baby's ability to eat with utensils, and fingers, too! For specific brand recommendations for first spoons, see appendix, page 215.

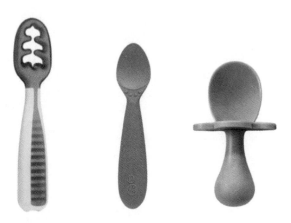

Left to right: NumNum GOOtensil, ezpz Tiny Spoon,
Grabease Ergonomic Spoon

How to Prepare First Foods

Research shows that you can offer almost any kind of food that you and the rest of the family are eating if items are soft, squishable, and easily adapted for baby's skill level. Cut foods into strips the width of an adult's pinky finger so that baby can use the palmer grasp (gripping the food in their little fist) and mouth the end. Examples include strips of avocado, ripe pears, and ripe banana. Babies also use a raking motion with their fingers to rake up smaller pieces of food, like smashed blueberries. This raking movement will emerge as an immature pincer grasp in the seventh month, where baby attempts to use the index finger and thumb to pinch food and bring it to the mouth. But that grasp takes time to master, and we don't expect kids to have it perfected until about 12 months of age. Offer both safe strips and pea-size soft foods for baby to practice and perfect in the first year.

Some believe that starting with anything but vegetables will predispose their baby to a sweet tooth. Research indicates that introducing vegetables first may be beneficial, but larger studies need to be conducted to make that a hard-and-fast rule. The most important guideline is to offer variety from the start. Rather than choosing one food group, try not to omit food groups. Learning to love all kinds of foods is due to *exposure* to all kinds of foods. Don't give up! Keep exposing your baby to a variety of foods, in small amounts. One tablespoon is the perfect serving size for these tiny samplings of new foods. Typically, a tablespoon is consumed in multiple bites or presentations. Remember, baby's mouth is small and can't handle a large amount all at once, so offer tiny tastes of that portion.

Tips & Tricks: Help Baby Grasp Slippery Foods

Put a teaspoon of bread crumbs in a jar or plastic bag and add pieces of safe, soft foods, like roasted squash. Give it a shake and coat the food strip for less slip and better grip. Other ideas for coating include almond flour, infant cereal, dried banana flakes, or a touch of roughly ground flax or a small sprinkling of chia seeds. Flax and chia are wonderful sources of nutrition, but too much can cause loose stool. Some feeding specialists prefer to grind small seeds like chia until children are about 9 months of age to ensure that none are accidentally inhaled while baby is still learning to coordinate the timing of chewing and swallowing. Use your best judgment and observe baby's oral skills to decide what's best for you. Try a crinkle cutter, which creates a wavelike texture or "crinkle" that is easy for baby's fingers to grasp.

Foods to Avoid Before Age One

There is certainly a large variety in all the food groups that you may serve your baby from the beginning if given in a safe shape and texture. There are a few things babies need to avoid before one year of age (one year corrected if your baby was born prematurely, see the box on page 59):

1. **Honey:** Infant botulism, a condition in which bacterial spores multiply to create a toxin, has been associated with honey. Avoid giving honey before baby is 12 months old and be mindful of honey as an added ingredient in recipes or packaged food products.

2. **Milk, as a beverage:** You learned earlier that breast milk or formula should provide most of a baby's nutrient needs before one year of age. Other than small sips of water offered at mealtimes, breast milk or formula should be the only liquid baby gets, to prevent conditions such as iron deficiency. Dairy foods, such as small amounts of cheese, yogurt, or cream found in recipes, are fine to offer your baby.

3. **Added salt:** Like the gastrointestinal tract, your baby's kidneys continue to grow and develop day by day. The kidneys, in the infant stage, are too immature to process added salt, so it is important to avoid this ingredient if serving your baby family meals. Also be mindful of processed, packaged foods that may contain excess sodium. Examples include certain breads, pasta sauces, soy sauces, and canned goods.

4. **Added sugar:** Though this ingredient isn't necessarily harmful in the same way that honey is to a baby, try not to include this in their daily routine. Sugar doesn't provide any beneficial calories for growth and development. Be mindful of added sugar as an ingredient in many packaged foods marketed for babies, including flavored "baby yogurts," and instead focus on offering a balance of whole foods. For best overall health, it is recommended that a parent wait to give their child added sugar until two years of age.[25]

5. **Juice, unless for medical reasons:** Fruit juice offers no nutritional benefits to your baby and has been shown to contain concerning amounts of arsenic and lead. Juice is mostly water and sugar.[26] Juice consumption in children is associated with dental cavities, nutritional imbalances, and diarrhea.[27] Occasionally, your pediatrician may recommend juice for medical reasons. For example, full-strength prune, apple, or pear juice may be used to treat constipation. Store-bought juice should be pasteurized, and homemade juices should be consumed immediately after blending.

6. **Deli meats, raw or undercooked eggs or meats, and unpasteurized cheeses:** Although it's rare, young babies can become very ill from listeriosis, a potentially serious disease caused by bacteria found in contaminated foods. Deli meats, pâté, undercooked poultry, and even side dishes or salads that have been exposed to the bacteria while stored at the deli counter are the most common culprits.[28] Raw or undercooked eggs, poultry, and meats pose a risk to anyone,

but babies are at a much higher risk for food poisoning due to E. coli and salmonella. Avoid offering homemade mayonnaise, hollandaise sauce, or other raw delicacies to babies and young children.

Babies under the age of six months should never have fresh spinach, beets, green beans, or carrots, due to the risk of a blood disorder caused by high nitrate levels in these foods. After six months, babies have enough stomach acid to tolerate these foods. As with any food, the key is to rotate variety on a daily basis, but you may choose to limit the quantities that you offer if you're concerned.

Restricting Foods

For babies under the age of one, remember that not offering sugar, as recommended by the AAP and other health organizations, is best for their body and brain health. Keep in mind that babies have no idea that you're not giving them foods with added sugar and won't miss it if they have never experienced it. If you'd like to include a "smash cake" on the first birthday and of course snap some pictures for lasting memories, please do! Does it need to be a grocery store cake with inches of frosting? Not necessarily, but it's always your choice! Perhaps bake or buy one that has only a thin schmear of frosting or that first taste of whipped cream instead. All the friends at the party, kids and adults alike, will enjoy it, too!

Heavy Metals in Store-Bought Purees and Other Foods

Heavy metals can seriously harm any child's brain and nervous system, especially babies and toddlers. Metals such as arsenic, lead, cadmium, or mercury have been shown to be present in store-bought purees and solid foods such as larger fish (e.g., shark, albacore or white tuna, swordfish) and in grains, especially the arsenic found in rice. These natural elements are found in the water and soil used to grow and harvest crops that are later pureed into baby food or sold as whole foods, like apples, sweet potatoes, and common fruit or vegetables that bring a vast source of nutrition as well. How then, can a parent limit their child's exposure to toxic metals in food and in the child's environment?[29]

The AAP recommends parenting proactively and taking the following food and environmental precautions[30]:

Food precautions

- **Consider making your own baby food.** Heavy metals can also get into food from manufacturing and packaging.

- **Breastfeed when possible.** Breastfeeding, rather than formula feeding, also can help reduce exposure to metals.

- **Make healthy fish choices.** Many fish are excellent sources of protein and other nutrients children need, and are still low in mercury. Choose light tuna (sometimes referred to as skipjack or yellowfin tuna), salmon, cod, whitefish, or pollock.

- **Variety is always key, and remember to wash well.** Fruits, vegetables, grains, and beans should be washed in cool water before prepping and serving.

- **Switch up your grains.** The AAP encourages fortified infant cereals to ensure varied nutrition for baby, but don't rely on just rice cereal. Rice cereal used to be the first choice when previous generations were feeding their infants, but the AAP has since changed its recommendations. Because rice tends to be higher in arsenic than other similar crops, it's best to limit rice instead, and the AAP specifically notes to include grains like "oats, barley, couscous, quinoa, farro and bulgur. Multi-grain infant cereals can be a good choice. Try to avoid using rice milk and brown rice syrup, which is sometimes used as a sweetener in processed toddler foods."[31] Brown rice tends to be higher in arsenic than white, but both should be limited. The AAP offers this tip when preparing rice of any kind: "When making rice from scratch, rinse it first. Cook it in extra water and then drain off the excess when it's done."[32]

- **Choose organic when possible.** Note that, even with organic foods, heavy metals may still be present, because processing and packaging contribute to the contaminant levels in the food.

Environmental precautions

- **Don't smoke or vape.** Even thirdhand smoke is dangerous to children. Regular and e-cigarettes may expose your child to cadmium and lead.

- **Address lead hazard in your home.** Peeling and chipping pain from older homes is the most common source of lead.

- **Test your water.** Contact your local health department to learn how to have your water tested.

Introducing Allergenic Foods without Fear

The thought of your child having an allergic reaction to a new food is frightening! However, thanks to recent groundbreaking research, medical professionals now understand the importance of introducing allergenic foods (like peanut butter, for example) *early and often* so that your child has less of a risk of developing an allergy. The "Top Nine,"[33] or the most common culprits for causing food allergies, are listed in the box that follows and may be introduced as soon as your child is ready to begin solids.

Generally, these foods should be introduced by themselves or mixed with another food your baby has ingested in the past. A good example of this is peanut butter, which should not be introduced alone because it is so sticky that it becomes a potential choking hazard. Instead, an easy way to introduce it is by mixing a small amount into a fruit puree or infant cereal. Eggs are another common allergen in infants and children. In fact, 1 to 8 percent of children are allergic to eggs. Eggs can be introduced in a variety of ways including baked into muffins or breads. If you think your child may be at higher risk of food allergy due to family history or severe eczema, it is best to talk to your medical provider about a safe plan of action for introduction. Here is a comprehensive list of how to introduce the allergens.

Top Nine Food Allergens	Ways to Introduce to Baby
Dairy	Breast milk, cow, or other animal milk incorporated into other recipes*, yogurt, cheeses *Not given as a beverage before 1 year of age
Eggs	Scrambled, egg bakes, frittatas, store-bought powders to be mixed into purees (brand examples: Lil Mixins; Ready, Set, Foods!)
Peanuts	Peanut butter mixed into fruit/vegetable/infant cereal puree, spread thinly on a slice of toast, mixed into baked goods like muffins or pancakes Note: Do not give peanuts in whole nut or nut butter form by itself to your baby, as these are both choking hazards.
Tree Nuts	Examples include almonds, hazelnuts, walnuts. Introduce in the same manner as peanuts.
Sesame	Tahini introduced in the same manner as other nuts Sesame seeds mixed into puree or another dish
Soy	Tofu, tempeh, natto Mashed, cooked edamame Note: Soy sauce is high in sodium, so use sparingly or not at all.
Wheat	Bread products, oats
Fish[34]	Fresh or frozen options cooked to at least 145°F (63°C)
Shellfish[35]	Fresh or frozen options cooked to at least 145°F (63°C). Chop finely and mix into moist foods

Allergic Reactions versus Food Intolerances

Watch for signs of an allergic reaction and notify your pediatrician immediately. Call 911 first if your baby presents with any of the following: hives; wheezing or trouble breathing; rash or itchy, red skin; swelling anywhere on the face or body; sudden stomach distress like vomiting or diarrhea; difficulty swallowing; dizziness; sudden lethargy; or unconsciousness. An allergic reaction can be life threatening. A mild allergic reaction does not appear to be too uncomfortable is still notable because the immune response can rapidly escalate and be deadly the next time. Food intolerances, in contrast, are not an immune response and are not life threatening; they typically include gastrointestinal symptoms like bloating or diarrhea.

Premature Babies May Need to Wait

Premature babies may need extra time to develop readiness for solid foods. Not all do, but consider discussing your preemie's needs with your pediatrician. When a baby is born early, feeding specialists can provide strategies on how to support immature gross- and fine-motor skills, allowing your child to start solids sooner rather than later. Part of the decision involves calculating corrected or adjusted age to account for the time difference between when your baby was born and a full-term birth. Adjusted age is the infant's actual age minus the number of weeks of prematurity. For example, a six-month-old baby who is born two months early may have the growth and development of a four-month-old. This adjustment to account for developmental milestones may extend to age two. If your baby was born prematurely, be sure to check with your pediatrician or other medical team members before starting solid foods. Each child is unique, and this decision is best discussed with your medical professional.[36]

Common Concerns

Baby isn't eating enough.

Babies intuitively know how much energy they require to grow, so the best thing you can do as a parent is to honor your baby's cues when it comes to the amount they can eat. Tiny samples, about a tablespoon, are less about consuming the food than exploring the sensory properties—the texture, subtle temperatures, and the aroma! These are critical months for kids to learn with all of their senses and reflexes, even if the amount consumed seems small compared to breastfeeding or bottle-feeding. Some babies will consume the average portion at 6 months of age and others might eat much more. Start with offering the tiny samples and if baby indicates the desire for more, offer a little bit more. Try not to get caught up in volume consumed or comparing your baby's eating habits to another baby. Focus on just one meal at a time and the joy in being together. Watch for more discussion on portion sizes as baby approaches their first birthday in chapter three (page 109).

My baby doesn't seem ready.

Talk to your pediatrician and bring this book to your next appointment. When parents come armed with knowledge about feeding development, the conversation easily shifts from "Don't worry, give it more time" to "You seem concerned, and it's great that you're doing your research. Let's get your baby some extra support to help both of you enjoy this experience." Your pediatrician may refer you to an experienced feeding professional, such as a speech-language pathologist, registered dietitian, or occupational therapist. The type of professional that's best suited to help your family will depend on what signs of readiness your baby is or is not demonstrating at the time.

My baby is gagging a lot!

In the next chapter, we'll explore gagging versus choking in detail. Gagging is typical for babies who are first being introduced to solid foods. Remember to start with the safe shapes and appropriate portion sizes. Many babies will benefit from purees for a few days before introducing handheld foods. If your baby continues to gag but doesn't appear distressed, see page 63 for more tips. If your baby appears to be uncomfortable and upset, stop solids for about a week and gently try again later. Bring any concerns to your baby's primary care provider just in case this is a medical issue and not simply your baby needing a bit more time to mature and develop feeding skills. If baby had a true choking episode, notify your pediatrician today, rather than waiting for the next well-child visit at the office.

My baby isn't progressing.

Take a video and share it with your pediatrician to explore all the possible reasons that baby isn't progressing. You may need to take a brief pause for a week before starting again. Sometimes a rest, allowing for an extra week of maturation, is all baby needs.

Nobody ever told me any of this!

Are any of the above concepts new to you? Perhaps some are the exact *opposite* of what you've read or been taught. I find that feeding myths abound not only online and on social media platforms, but unfortunately even in some medical professionals' offices. Let's look at some of the most common myths about this stage of feeding development and how they can be debunked.

Feeding Myths

My baby will lose weight if I don't start solids soon.

Apart from a brief period immediately after birth, weight loss is *never* something normally seen in babies and toddlers. If your child is experiencing weight loss, it might be a red flag for an underlying condition that needs to be investigated with the help of your medical team. While a registered dietitian can help you choose nutrient-dense food options when your baby requires more energy to grow, starting solids should never be solely for the sake of helping your baby gain weight, since their weight may be due to other medical issues.

Starting solids early will help baby sleep through the night.

As much as 46 percent of parents believe that starting solids will help their baby sleep longer at night.[37] The hope, of course, is that the poor parents would be able to get more sleep! Unfortunately, no research proves this to be true, and it's not worth the risk to introduce solids when baby isn't developmentally ready.

Babies need teeth to eat.

At 6 months of age, many babies don't yet have any teeth. The teeth that do pop through the gums first were never really designed for chewing food. It's the big molars toward the back of your child's mouth that grind tougher food, and those don't come in until toddlerhood. Imagine the window of opportunity lost if you waited to introduce solid foods until your child had become a toddler! Babies don't need teeth to eat, they need safe foods like steamed carrots and strips of avocado toast to gum, smush, and swallow. This early practice builds the foundation to break down the chewier foods when they are older and they have the teeth to do it!

Offering purees and handheld solids at the same time increases the risk of choking.

For typically developing babies, there is no need to separate the two textures as long as kids aren't trying to manage a bite of puree in the middle of a bite of handheld solids. Even adults would cough on that unexpected combination! One bite at a time, please. Likewise, save foods like soup (thin liquids with chunks of safe solids) for the toddler years, or better yet, blend the entire soup into one texture for your baby. As a pediatric feeding specialist, I have 20 years of experience and advanced training in hospital and home settings, helping babies with motor and medical challenges. For those children, a parent might offer purees alone at one meal and safe solids at another as baby learns to manipulate each separately, one at a time.

Babies learn to chew first, and swallow later.

Infants learn to swallow while nestled in the womb, swallowing amniotic fluid. They experience flavor first via amniotic fluid and next via breast milk or formula, coordinating the suck-swallow-breathe sequence in preparation for their first taste of solid foods. When solids are introduced, some of it is swallowed, and some is pushed out of the mouth due to the tongue-protrusion reflex. Only then do they start to chew, beginning by mashing their tongue and eventually by munching up and down with their gums. The rotary chew, where the jaw moves in a more circular fashion, then emerges but is not mastered until age two. So, babies learn to swallow first and eventually chew, and by age three learn to eat all kinds of textures.

If baby spits out food, that means they don't like it.

There are so many reasons that babies spit out food! One possibility is that the taste is overwhelming, too hot, or too spicy, and parents will need to adjust accordingly. It's possible they don't care for it, but exposure to all sorts of tastes takes time and repetition. Most often, when infants expel food, it's because they are still learning to control the tongue-protrusion reflex, or they have a tongue-tie. Tethered oral tissues, most often found under the tongue (ankyloglossia or tongue-tie) or beneath the upper lip can impact a child's ability to manipulate food safely. When the tongue is restricted by a short or thick frenum (a strand of tissue found beneath the tongue and connecting to the floor of the mouth) mobility and proper placement for eating and speech can be an issue. These are just two of the most common types of tethered oral tissues that influence a child's willingness to continue to try new foods. If you suspect that your child is tongue- or lip-tied, consult with an orofacial myologist with advanced training in tethered oral tissues.

Offer small pieces only after baby has developed the pincer grasp.

Babies need small pieces of food to develop and fine-tune the pincer grasp. Offer both safely cut strips and handheld pieces of food along with smaller pieces for practice. Handheld pieces should be firm enough for baby to grasp but soft enough to bite off pieces to practice chewing and swallowing. Smaller pieces for pincer-grasp development should be the size of a pea and if possible, cut into a soft cube, making it easier to pick up. Examples of handhelds include strips of roasted sweet potato with no skin, sliced lasagna noodles, and very soft, moist meats that break apart into small pieces in the mouth. Examples of foods that support pincer-grasp development include cereals that melt easily with saliva, such as puffs or O-shaped cereals; cooked cubes of carrots (bags of peas and carrots from the freezer aisle are fabulous for this!); and moist chicken breast cut into tiny cubes. Toss tiny cubes of moist foods in bread crumbs or chia seeds to make them less slippery.

Chapter Two

Building Momentum & Communication Skills

• 6 TO 12 MONTHS •

How Babies Communicate

Now that your baby is 6 months old, they will be using a variety of gestures, facial expressions, babbling, laughing, and crying to communicate their wants and needs, and to indicate emotion. You, too, are changing the way you communicate: You may not even realize that you have been speaking a second language known as "motherese" to your baby. Researchers call it infant-directed speech, and it is a universal way that parents speak to their newborn and young babies. Instinctively, we slow our pace of speech, pause more, change our pitch, and exaggerate the vowels. A 2017 report from Princeton's Baby Lab[1] indicates that mothers unconsciously shift even their vocal timbre, or the unique quality of their own voice, just for baby. Why? Because babies love it, and no matter what language a parent is teaching their child, they learn language faster when parents speak to them in this universal manner. Babies are hardwired to pay attention to infant-directed speech. They learn to smile in response to your interactions, when upset they quiet down at the sound of your soothing voice and comforting embrace, and they coo back and forth with you. Yet most babies will not utter a first word until closer to their first birthday.

If babies are not yet saying words, how can they be learning language? The difference lies in the definition of speech versus language. According to the American Speech-Language-Hearing Association (ASHA), "Speech is how we say sounds and words" and "language refers to the words we use and how we use them to share ideas and get what we want."[2] Baby is developing two types of language: receptive and expressive. Receptive language refers to the understanding of what's said to us. Expressive language refers to our ability to share our own message with others, either via sign language, body language, verbalizations, or other forms of communication. When listening to the infant-directed speech of the parent, language is embedded in how the parent says the words. For baby, listening to speech builds language skills.

Babies learn speech and language not only by listening but also by looking at the parent's face, specifically the mouth, while the parent is speaking to the child. Imitation also plays a key role from any early age. Newborns have been found to imitate a parent's mouth movements as they gaze at the parent's face. All along, our everyday routines like breastfeeding and bottle-feeding have been contributing to speech and language development, right up to the day that your baby is introduced to solids.

Now that the foundation for communication is in place, what are the gestures, sounds, and body language that baby uses to talk to you from the end of the sixth month to the end of the eleventh month? According to ASHA,[3] during this time, baby will learn to:

- Turn and look in the direction of sounds.
- Look toward where you point.
- Turn when you call their name.
- Understand words for common items and people—like *cup, truck, juice,* and *daddy.*
- Start to respond to simple words and phrases, like "No," "Come here," and "Want more?"
- Play games with you, like peekaboo and pat-a-cake.
- Listen to songs and stories for a short time.

These skills refer to how your baby understands your gestures and words, or receptive language.

Expressive language, which includes speech sounds, refers to how baby expresses their understanding to others. According to ASHA,[4] during this time period, baby will learn to:

- Babble long strings of sounds, like *mimi upup babababa.*
- Use sounds and gestures to get and keep attention.
- Point to objects and show them to others.
- Use gestures like waving bye, reaching for "up," and shaking their head no.
- Imitate different speech sounds.
- Say one or two words, like *hi, dog, dada, mama,* or *uh-oh.* This will happen around their first birthday, but sounds may not be clear.

Your baby uses these newfound skills to participate in family mealtimes and other food experiences. Mindful communication is at the heart of responsive feeding and one of the primary ways that we bond with our children. Touch, gesture, and speech are all forms of language that help us express our love for each other and shared experiences, especially when it comes to food. In your child's first three years of life, you will feed and share the joy of food with your family more than 6,500 times! More than just opportunities to eat, each mealtime is an occasion to support your child's cognitive development and emotional health. Language is the richest component of that, whether expressed in a hug, first words, or as we tell stories around the dinner table.

Sign Language for Babies

Sign language is one form of gesturing that is rich with meaning and a popular second language to teach baby in the first year. Cari Ebert, an international expert and SLP specializing in children under three, shared these guidelines for signing with baby:

ADVICE FROM AN EXPERT SPEECH-LANGUAGE PATHOLOGIST

Mealtime is a wonderful opportunity to enhance language development! Manual signs can be introduced long before your child ever says their first words. Learning just a few signs can increase your child's functional communication skills, decrease frustration, and strengthen your relationship with your little one through positive and successful interactions.

When introducing signs, it is important to always say the word as you model the sign. There are three opportunities during mealtime when you can model signs for your language learner.

1. **When offering choices:** "Do you want an apple or a banana?" Ask the question while modeling the signs for *apple* and *banana*—then wait for your child to make a choice either by reaching for or looking at the desired item. Once a choice has been made, say just the word, and model the sign again. Wait to see if your child attempts to make the sign, too. After waiting 3 to 4 seconds, give your child the desired food regardless of their response or lack of response. Do not ever withhold food to coerce language. Model and move on with a smile.

2. **When your child is fussing:** A child who is crying or whining is communicating something important! At mealtime it is likely either a desire to eat and drink more or be finished.

Ask the question "Do you want more or are you all done?" while modeling the signs for *more* and *all done*. Eventually your child will use these signs (and eventually spoken words!) independently during mealtime. If baby is not yet ready to sign in return, interpret their body language to decide how to respond.

3. **To describe the mealtime experience:** You can say, "Red peppers are delicious" while modeling the sign for the color red. Or you can say, "You are using your spoon like a big kid" while modeling the sign for *spoon*. Get in the habit of using positive, descriptive language to bring more joy to the mealtime experience.

Here are some suggested first signs to introduce during mealtime and snack time: *eat, drink, milk, water, more, all done, spoon, open, hot*, and your child's preferred foods (*banana, apple, cracker, cereal*, and so on). Visit signingtime.com to build your signing vocabulary.

Eating Times & Growing Times

Your newborn may have been fed on demand, but in the first six months of life a natural schedule likely emerged as you began to interpret baby's hunger cues. Once baby has been introduced to solids and has had a few months of practice at least two times per day, you can slowly shift to a predictable feeding schedule and increase meals to three or four meals per day by age one. There's a crucial difference between "eating times" and "growing times": Eating times are when kids are offered food (about every two to two-and-a-half hours), and growing times are when kids play, learn, or rest.

By 12 months, kids should be on a predictable schedule to help them continue to pay attention to their own hunger cues and communicate their needs to you. The consistency of a feeding schedule helps children tune in to their own hunger and fullness cues. When kids are allowed to feel a reasonable amount of hunger, they tend to have more interest in trying new foods at meal and snack times. When kids graze throughout the day, there is no consistency, and they may be responding to feelings that have no relation to hunger, like boredom. If they're eating throughout the day, they are not attending to their own ability to self-regulate and recognize hunger versus satiety.

Feeding schedules and real life don't always align perfectly and may shift depending on the length of naps and growth spurts (when kids just seem hungrier than usual). Your knowledge of how your baby communicates will guide you to a schedule that works for you and baby—and will be the foundation for how and when you offer meals and snacks.[5] Before baby's first birthday, you will find yourself offering "mini meals" more often than true snacks. (Snacks are typically much smaller than meals, but mini meals are bigger than snacks.) However, the rest of the family will be following the meal and snack rotation, and it's ideal to bring baby to the table with the family at mealtime, or for the occasional mini meal for baby while everyone else is enjoying a smaller snack.

The World Health Organization (WHO) recommends that you offer solids two or three times per day for children 6 to 8 months of age, and three or four solid meals for babies and toddlers after the age of 9 months. Offer a few teaspoons or tablespoons of foods from various food groups throughout each meal. If baby indicates that they would like more, offer more. After the age of one, snack time will be a consistent part of your child's hunger schedule.

Tipping the Scales from Liquids to Solids

Stacy Zimmels, a London-based pediatric SLP and lactation consultant (IBCLC), suggests that parents imagine a set of balanced weighing scales as baby transitions from breastfeeding or bottle-feeding to gradually eating more solid foods.

ADVICE FROM AN EXPERT LACTATION CONSULTANT

Imagine one side of the scale empty and the opposite side weighed down with breast milk or formula. Gradually, solid food is added to balance out the volume or weight of the liquids. Zimmels emphasizes that "the speed at which those scales shift and the point at which the balance tips is really very dependent on each individual baby." Milk is typically offered before one or two tastings of solid food per day. Once a second tasting is added, Zimmels recommends moving breastfeeding or bottle-feeding slightly further away from the offerings of solids, but still keeping those milk feedings before the meal.

Once baby begins to chew and swallow solids with relative ease, they will likely begin to reduce the milk they take in, and the imaginary scales will begin to shift. "For bottle-fed infants, you may notice that they drop an ounce or two from one or more of their bottles or that they drop a large amount from one bottle at a certain time of the day," says Zimmels. "Breastfeeding infants may reduce the length of time and/or frequency of breastfeeds. Follow their lead with this. Once a bottle gets to around two or three ounces at any one feed you can stop offering it and move the mealtimes a little closer to each other."

If your infant doesn't naturally reduce their milk intake very much, then Zimmels suggests the following options: If they are progressing with their eating skills and the volumes, you can continue to follow their lead. However, if they are not, especially if they are formula feeding, then you can reduce the amount of milk you offer them. This can either be by cutting out a whole bottle or reducing the volumes in each or in a few selected bottles gradually by an ounce at a time. It's always a good idea to talk to your pediatrician about this plan to ensure adequate hydration and nutrition.

For nursing mothers, the shift to solid foods may be a slower process, and the timing of nursing may be the solution. Consider breastfeeding after meals rather than before. Zimmels shared that for some mothers working outside the home, keeping up with pumping is challenging and you may wish to reduce it. However, if your pumping schedule is working for you, you can maintain a little more breast milk in the diet for the immunological benefits it continues to provide and start by being more flexible with timings of bottles and solid meals.[6]

One Family, One Meal:
Safe Foods to Offer

I am a strong believer in the concept of one family, one meal! When a parent can prepare one meal for the entire family (perhaps adapting certain textures for the safety of babies and toddlers), it benefits everyone. Parents have less mealtime prep and planning overall, and children are exposed to more variety. When the whole family has the same foods on their plates, parents are modeling healthy eating habits, chewing skills for baby, and the enjoyment of all kinds of food.

In this section, you'll find three charts. The first includes a few examples of typical recipes that you can serve to the entire family and often to your baby, too, with some slight modifications in how you cut or serve the ingredients. The second includes a list of whole foods and nutritious foods from your pantry that you can offer your baby. As long as you consider the size of their airway and how well their gums can break down the food, you'll be able to decide which of the foods you enjoy are also safe for baby. Remember to refer to the short list in chapter one regarding foods to avoid (see page 72) but in general, my two hard-and-fast rules are:

1. Can baby break it down completely with their gums?
2. How likely is this to lodge in baby's airway if they lose control of the food?

The ability to break the food apart with the lateral margins (sides) of the gumline is impressive in babies! They are remarkably strong, and chewing on appropriate foods only helps to build the musculature they need for chewy, dense foods like steak or bagels when they are older. On one hand, we want baby to be able to break down the food with a chewing motion before swallowing it. On the other hand, that same jaw can clamp down hard on a strip of flank steak and rip off a piece, leaving a chunk of meat that is now impossible to chew without teeth. If baby's tongue-thrust reflex, which is already beginning to fade, doesn't push the meat out, baby will likely gag as it approaches the back of the throat. The gag isn't foolproof. If I sound like an alarmist, then please consider the second question.

How likely is this piece of food to lodge in baby's airway? In the BLISS study (a commonly cited randomized control trial intended to examine the likelihood of choking when parents followed a modified BLW approach), one result may surprise you. "A total of 35 percent of infants choked at least once between 6 and 8 months of age, and there were no significant group differences in the number of choking events at any time." In other words, more than a third of all the participating babies choked, no matter what feeding model their parents followed.

In my work with parents, the foods I suggest are more conservative than you may find elsewhere. I've even seen recommendations that babies chew on large strips of steak or a turkey leg at 7 months old. The idea is that baby can mouth the pieces of meat and suck the juices. If you're 100 percent certain that the meat you offer baby cannot be broken down or bitten off into a chunk that would block the airway, then go for it. One of the general principles taught to the parents in the BLISS study who were following a modified BLW method was to "test foods before they were offered to ensure they were soft enough to mash on the roof of the mouth . . . or are large and fibrous enough that small pieces do not break off when sucked and chewed (e.g., strips of meat)."

Even with these guidelines, which are the same guidelines I am presenting to you in this book, one third of the children choked. The infants were able to resolve the choking episode on their own about half the time. Choking was defined as full or partial blockage of the airway, affecting breathing.

My point? No matter what method of feeding you choose, it is not uncommon for babies to choke. Reduce that risk by offering safe solids, cut appropriately according to texture and babies' skill. Offer purees as yet another texture for baby to learn from, but don't linger there. Variety, in safe forms, is essential. Always sit with baby while they are eating and keep an eye on them. You don't need to be face-to-face, but maintain your attention to ensure that if baby does choke, you're able to respond immediately. Because you've been practicing responsive feeding, your experience observing your baby's communication signals and body language will be an added benefit.

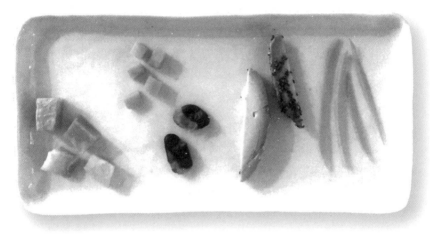

Cooked or soft squishable foods, from left to right: large cubes (cheese), small cubes (cheese), smashed (beans), pinky-strips (avocado with chia seeds), matchsticks (raw carrot)

Five Ways to Cut Food for Your Baby

The types of foods to offer baby may vary, but there are five ways to cut food for baby to grasp and bring to the mouth, whether on a utensil or directly from their hands.

1. **Matchsticks:** Slivers of foods that can be broken down when baby bites down on them can still provide a satisfying crunch! Try matchsticks of skinless raw apples, pears, or blanched carrots.

2. **Pinky-strips:** Many foods can be offered in strips, about the size of an adult pinky finger. (If you've got big hands like me, your pinky might be wider than most. Adjust accordingly!) Offer pinky-strips of soft foods that baby can gnaw and still manage small pieces that break off. Stick to moist foods like strips of roasted zucchini or avocado, or roasted fruits like pears and apples.

3. **Smashed:** A quick "smush" on a round food like a cooked bean will assure safety yet allow baby to pick it up with ease. Smashed foods can also be presented on a preloaded utensil for self-feeding, directly from a parent's fingers, or while holding the utensil for baby.

4. **Small cubes:** Cubes are terrific for babies because they are ideal for learning to use the pincer grasp. The edges can be detected inside the mouth much more easily. compared to smoother foods. Cut soft cubes into pea-size for any age, and never offer hard cubes (e.g., parmesan cheese) that could lodge in baby's trachea if accidently swallowed whole.

5. **Large cubes:** Children who have an emerging pincer grasp and are at least 9 months of age can begin to try soft cubes about the size of a cherry tomato. Unlike a tomato or grape, the cube should always be compressible with little force, even if just compressed between the tongue and the palate. Remember, whole grapes and cherry tomatoes should be quartered until age four, and these larger cubes are soft and squishable. When cubes are that soft, should one be swallowed whole, it is likely to be expelled quickly or squished from the musculature force of the swallow. It's not comfortable to swallow large cubes, as anyone knows who has swallowed a bite of food that was inadequately chewed, but it isn't likely to be choked on. Why, then, would we not offer larger cubes to younger babies? The less experienced baby is more likely to swallow a large,

soft cube whole and experience frequent discomfort. It's best to wait until these emerging eaters have learned more advanced chewing skills via the motor window described earlier in this book.

How to Prepare Each Food Group

No matter how you decide to prep foods for baby, remember these two rules:

1. Can baby break it down completely with their gums?

2. How likely is this to lodge in baby's airway if they lose control of the food?

Fruits and vegetables: These can be cut into pinky-strips or age-appropriate safe-size pieces. Raw, hard, or round chunks of fruits or vegetables should be avoided until after age four. See tips on how to soften foods quickly before serving on page 78 and the earlier illustration on pinky-strips and cubes. Ripe fruits (such as watermelon or very soft pears) that are already soft and squishable against the tongue and hard palate do not need to be softened via cooking.

Meats: Fibrous strips of steak are sometimes recommended as one way to introduce meat to babies as young as 6 months. However, it's important to clarify that thick, fibrous steaks are not something adults enjoy, and it's more likely that families will serve tender meats to their families. When serving tender meats, limit portions to moist pea-size bites for baby or finely chopped soft meats mixed with a sauce for easier manipulation for chewing and swallowing. After the age of 9 months, pinky-strips of succulent meats may be offered with close supervision. Be sure baby has swallowed completely before offering more, because meats can lodge in the space between the gums and the cheeks (the lateral sulci) and become gummier with time. Always check the roof of baby's mouth after meals or before laying baby down to sleep to make sure no gummy foods like bread or meat have stuck to the hard palate, especially behind the front gums. Another option is to offer the thick bone from your steak with the large pieces of meat trimmed away. The shreds of meat that are still attached to the bone are a wonderful way for baby to enjoy the flavor with a bit of texture without risking a choking incident. The large bone serves as the perfect handle for little fists to grasp as they explore the flavor.

Grains: Small pieces of grains can be frustrating for young babies to manage in their mouth, because they're difficult to gather into a bolus (the portion of food we swallow) and propel backward to swallow. But too large a portion is also hard to manipulate because the grains spread so easily into the nooks and crannies of the gums and cheeks. The best way to serve grains is to add a bit of oily dressing or smooth dairy product (plain yogurt or a soft cheese like goat cheese) to the grains. Soft tofu mixed in is another easy way to make grains silky and manageable. This makes it easier for babies to lick off their hands and fingers and it tends to stick better to utensils. The added moisture also makes it easier to bind together in the mouth for comfortable swallowing. When offering a portion from your fingers or via a preloaded utensil, keep the amount small enough that it won't overwhelm baby. Large globs of grains, if packed tightly, could cause choking. Breads and muffins are best served in small cubes, unless toasted. Larger cubes of breads can be difficult for babies in their first year to manage safely. Lightly toasting strips or small cubes of bread is ideal because the added texture is less likely to gum up in the mouth and the rougher texture is easier for the tongue to locate. As long as the crust isn't too thick, it's fine to leave it on the strip of toast.

Dairy: Prior to age one, babies should not be consuming "milk" beverages other than breast milk or formula, and that includes milk alternatives (e.g., rice milk, soy milk, almond milk). As reported by the Academy of Nutrition and Dietetics, "Cow's milk, soy milk, rice milk and homemade formulas are not appropriate for babies during the first year because they have the wrong ratio of protein, fat and carbohydrate"[7] and many have added sugars. Most are missing important nutrients for health, growth, and development. Milk-based soups or sauces are best avoided until after age one. However, small amounts of soft pasteurized cheese, yogurt, or any dairy baked into recipes are fine to offer your baby. Nondairy substitutes such as silken tofu or coconut-milk yogurts are fabulous options, too.

How to Soften Foods Quickly

Steaming: The great thing about steaming foods is that it's quick and can be done in less than fifteen minutes. Place a few inches of water in a saucepan and add a steamer basket. Chop or slice foods while the water is heating to a boil. Add the foods to the steamer basket, cover and check frequently for the ideal stage of softness. To cool quickly, drain the water and add the foods to an ice bath (described in the next section). Pat dry before serving to baby.

Blanching: Even quicker than steaming, blanching provides moisture to foods like raw carrots, broccoli, or apples without sacrificing the crunch. Remember to serve these types of foods in matchstick form. For older kids, we'll discuss ways to blanch bigger pieces later in this book. Cover the chopped fruits or vegetables with an inch of boiling water or just enough to cover them. While the water is getting hot, prepare a small bowl of equal parts water and ice. Boil the pieces for one to two minutes or until you can easily pierce them with a fork. Drain and immediately plunge into the ice bath to stop the cooking process. Although firm to hold, a blanched matchstick's texture when baby bites into it is consistent with spaghetti cooked al dente, but with a subtle crunch. Pat dry before serving to baby in matchstick form. Larger pieces can be stored in a container in the refrigerator and will stay moist for 24 hours. Add a slightly damp paper towel in the container to make them last a few days longer.

One Meal, One Family: Quick Prep & Set Aside for Baby

The chart below offers examples from each food group to offer to children 6 months and older. Whether you're using an ingredient as part of a larger casserole or just want a fresh, whole food option to give to baby during the family meal, I hope this list will spur your imagination and help you consider all the possibilities when it comes to preparing wholesome food quickly for your little one.

Soft, Ripe Fruits	Soft, Cooked Vegetables	Grains	Cooked Proteins	Dairy or Similar Dairy Substitutes
Avocado	Broccoli	Barley	Soft beans (smushed)	Soft pasteurized cheeses (as spreads)
Apple	Carrots	Breads & Muffins	Eggs	
Banana	Mushrooms	Buckwheat	Some fish	Semi-hard cheeses (in tiny, pea-size cubes only and squished slightly)
Kiwi	Parsnips	Couscous	Meats	
Melon	Peas	Crackers (ones that melt with saliva only, like fish crackers)	Nuts or Seeds Butters	
Pear	Sweet Potatoes		Tofu	
Strawberries	Zucchini	Quinoa		

One Meal, One Family: Quick Tips for Main Dishes for Babies and Young Toddlers

Family Recipe	Puree Option	Mashed Option	Finger Food Option	Self-Feeding or Parent Feeding Utensil Options
Lasagna	Puree meat, cheese, and sauce after cooking	Mash entire piece	Slice noodles into strips	Provide child-safe utensil for dipping or preloaded
Chili—reserve some before adding spices that add heat for these adaptations	Puree chili after cooking	Spoon out beans, meat, and veggies and mash, adding liquid as needed	Bits of meat, beans, and vegetables	Smash and pierce beans or smash onto child-safe utensil
Omelet, quiche, or frittata	Chop finely and stir in butter or melted cheese to create puree	Mash with fork	Pinky-strips or small cubes	Pierce, scoop, or smash onto child-safe utensil
Pizza	Puree sauce, soft veggies, or meats and cheese	Mash toppings and sauce with fork	Offer strips of soft (not crispy) crust and small cubes of safely cut toppings.	Pierce or smash toppings onto child-safe utensil

One Meal, One Family: Quick Tips for Simple Side Dishes for Babies and Young Toddlers

Family Recipe	Puree Option	Mashed Option	Finger Food Option	Self-Feeding or Parent Feeding Utensil Options
Sweet Potato	Boil or roast, then puree	Mash with fork	Cooked Pinky-strips or small cubes	Pierce or smash onto child-safe utensil
Carrot	Boil or roast, then puree	Mash cooked carrots with fork	Cooked Pinky-strips or small cubes of carrots	Pierce or smash onto child-safe utensil
Avocado	Mash avocado with olive oil, plain yogurt, and/or lemon juice to thin into a puree	Mash instead of using blender	Slices of avocado rolled in chia seeds or cracker crumbs for added nutrition and less slip	Pierce, scoop, or smash onto child-safe utensil
Roasted potatoes or fries	Puree gently, using a hand blender, with olive oil, coconut oil, or butter to prevent gummy texture	Mash with fork	Wedges, larger chunks, and fries are good options if potato is softer and not too crispy	Pierce or smash onto child-safe utensil

One Meal, One Family at the Table

Pull baby's feeding chair up to your family table and ditch the high-chair tray as soon as possible. Baby will reap the benefits, and you'll have less mess. Baby has a wider surface for food to rest, resulting in less food ending up on the floor. Family mealtimes aren't just about the meal; it's where we connect as a family. When baby is truly at the table with the rest of the family, they are more likely to be part of the conversation. In my book *Adventures in Veggieland*, I shared that "research has demonstrated that a routine that includes daily mealtimes plays a crucial role in language development for children. Both expressive and receptive language skills improve when children are part of the mealtime table with their parents and older siblings, and those mealtime conversations also seem to influence early reading skills."[8] Just like the high chair tray, the tabletop should align just above the lowest rib, so that baby can easily rest their elbows on the table for added stability.

The Right Tools in Little Hands: Utensils, Cups & Plates

From the day you introduce solid foods, your baby can also be introduced to small utensils and cups. Raised plates and bowls that suction to the tray or table are ideal, because baby can grasp the side of the bowl with one hand for added stability while self-feeding with the other hand. Food placed directly on the tray is easy—just be sure to clean the entire surface well between feedings.

Right-Size Pre-Spoons

Pre-spoons are typically flat and sometimes textured dippers with short, squat handles for little fists to grab. The shorter handle might also be textured for better grip or be shaped in an ergonomic fashion to position baby's grip correctly as their motor skills continue to develop. I always offer these first as children are learning to dip and turn the utensil up to the mouth. But they make great utensils for young toddlers, too, especially those with smaller hands and mouths, like some preemies. Kids first learn to "dip and flip the wrist" to bring the pre-spoon (often upside down) to their mouths. Toddlers learn to scoop with more control and without spilling before rotating the wrist to place the utensil in the mouth. Progressing from a dipper or pre-spoon to a spoon with a deeper spoon bowl aligns with the development of the dip, scoop, and controlled wrist rotation. I'll share tips on how to boost that refined skill in chapter four (page 127).

Right-Size Spoons and Forks

The handle of your child's spoon and fork is just as important as the end that goes into the mouth. For children up to age 18 months, choose a utensil that has a short, fat handle or that is short and slightly curved in the middle. Thin, longer-handled spoons are meant for adult hands, when a parent is doing the spoon-feeding. Still, because babies love to participate, I often feed them with the shorter-handled option in case they'd like a turn, too! Some spoons and forks have choke-shields, which serve two purposes. First, the shield helps to prevent babies who are just learning to direct a utensil into their mouth from shoving it in too far and eliciting a gag and/or possibly pushing food too far back before chewing. Second, the shield sets them up for success by directing their fist into that "just right'" position for holding their own utensil.

Spoon-Feeding Tips

If you are feeding your baby with a spoon, the way you present the spoon can help them develop better lip and tongue control. The trick is to teach baby to do what comes most naturally to them— sucking the food off the spoon. This helps position their tongue in the correct position for learning to self-feed, too.

Try your best to face your child, as close to eye level as possible. I'm very tall, so I tend to sit on a small stool when feeding kids in a high chair. Their little feet rest on my knees, and it's a sweet connection! Most important, my face is directly across from theirs so they can watch my mouth and my facial expressions, and I theirs.

Standing above baby or sitting much higher than them creates a choking hazard as baby extends their neck and chin to look up at you, making it more difficult to protect the airway. With each bite, that hyperextension can cause poorly controlled food to topple toward the back of the throat, and baby could aspirate or choke. Plus, it's just so uncomfortable to try to swallow in that position! When you're higher than baby, you're also more likely to lift the handle of the spoon upward, scraping the food on the roof of the mouth.

- Start with just the tip of the spoon dipped in smooth puree. Gradually move from a taste to a spoonful. This may take a few days to help baby feel comfortable, but if you choose a dipper or a spoon that is flat and small, you won't overwhelm them. (Refer to the appendix, page 215, for specific brands.)

- Allow baby to come to you. As discussed in chapter one, hold the spoon as if it were floating in the air. Allow your baby to initiate the bite, learning slightly forward or with a look of expectation, rather than you directing the spoon into the mouth simply because that little mouth was open. Once the spoon is in their mouth, pause and allow baby to close their lips on the spoon. The moment they close their lips, they will naturally and gently suck once on the spoon. That's your signal to pull the spoon straight out and dip it into the puree again.

- A common mistake is to lift up on the handle of the spoon, scraping the puree behind the alveolar ridge or the top, front gumlines. Depositing food there makes it stick to the roof of the mouth, causing baby to thrust their tongue and push the food back out. Between 6 and 12 months, the tongue-thrust reflex is intended to fade while baby learns to control tongue movements. By causing the tongue to repeatedly push forward due to food on the hard palate, we are interfering with the learning process. Instead, keep the spoon parallel to the floor, gliding it out in one smooth motion.

- Before offering more puree, allow time for baby to propel the puree backward and swallow. In six-month-olds, you may notice baby pushing the food back out a little bit and then swallowing. It's OK! That anterior-posterior movement is how baby has been using their tongue for breastfeeding and bottle-feeding and, solid foods require more posterior movement. They'll get the hang of it with practice.

A Spoon for Each Hand

Bring three spoons to the table. Babies like to grab anything you're offering, and that's a good thing to boost along self-feeding! Let baby have a spoon in each hand and use the third for offering puree or mashed foods. Mashed foods require a bit more oral skill than smooth purees, so I typically start with purees, but it's not essential. If you read baby's cues and offer tiny tastes rather than a big spoonful at first, you're being a responsive feeder.

Perfecting the Pincer Grasp

Babies first rake up food and use the palm of their hand to grasp it in little fists. Between 6 and 12 months, you'll notice more refined movements emerge as baby begins to practice the pincer grasp. Perfecting that OK symbol—where the thumb and the forefinger hold each piece with precision—takes time, but it's important to offer your child opportunities to practice. Try these five easy activities, and you'll notice your little one rapidly progressing!

1. Collect a few lids from baby food jars for this activity. Take an old oatmeal box, cut a slit in the lid, and show your child how to pick up the lids and drop them in the box.

2. During bath time, use rubber bath toys that squirt when squeezed with two fingers.

3. During mealtimes, hold a round piece of cereal in your own fingers, using a pincer grasp, and offer the cereal to your child. Hang onto it as they practice grabbing it with their thumb and forefinger.

4. Place one piece of cereal in a plastic "shot glass" or similar-size narrow container. The container should be approximately two inches tall and just wide enough for your child's thumb and forefinger to reach in and pull out the cereal.

5. While you're at the coffee shop, entertain your child by stringing three pieces of circular cereal on a coffee stirrer. Hold it perpendicular to the tabletop and let your child pull off the cereal pieces one by one using their thumb and forefinger.[9]

Learning to use a pincer grasp in a controlled manner leads to future success in many other life skills: holding a pencil in preschool; fastening snaps, zippers, and buttons; and even cutting with scissors. The same is true for learning to use utensils, which we'll see in chapter three (page 125).

Step Away from Spouted Sippy Cups

Back in January 2014, I wrote an article titled "Step Away from the Sippy Cup."[10] Posted on social media, it created a stir of emotions in parents ranging from "Glad I learned this today!" to "You're an idiot. My kid drank from a sippy cup and she still went to Harvard." (That comment was my favorite.)

Sippy cups became all the rage in the 1980s, along with oversize shoulder pads, MC Hammer parachute pants, and bangs that stood up like a waterspout on top of your head. A mechanical engineer, tired of their toddler's trail of juice throughout the house, set out to create a spill-proof cup that would "outsmart the child." Soon,

Playtex offered a licensing deal, and spouted sippy cups were marketed as a necessary next step before introducing an open cup or a straw cup. The American marketing machine has convinced a generation of parents that transitioning from breast or bottle to the sippy cup is part of the developmental process of eating. The problem is, sippy cups aren't necessary except to keep carpets clean, and those sippy cups seem to linger through preschool.

Sippy cups were invented for parents, not for kids. The next transition from breast and/or bottle is to learn to drink from a straw cup. An open cup can also be introduced at this time, but babies won't be able to drink from an open cup immediately. Most babies can learn to drink from a straw in one day. I suggest cutting down the straw so that the child can just get their lips around it but can't anchor their tongue underneath it. That's my issue with the sippy cup: It continues to promote the anterior-posterior movement of the tongue, characteristic of a suckle-like pattern that infants use for breastfeeding or bottle-feeding. Sippy cups limit the child's ability to develop a more mature swallowing pattern, especially with continued use after the first year. The spout blocks the tongue tip from rising to the alveolar ridge just above the front teeth and forces the child to continue to push their tongue forward and back as they suck on the spout to extract the juice.

When speech therapists assess oral motor development in babies and young children, we are looking for anything that would impact the child's ability to function at an age-appropriate level. The issue is that those sippy cups are carried in the car, left at day care, and seem to travel with the child on a daily basis. They tend to linger through preschool. Just like pacifier use, which should be limited after 6 months of age, the impact of spouted sippy cups may depend on frequency, duration, and intensity of the suck. Speech-language pathologists and dentists have observed that prolonged use can lead to incorrect tongue posture (how we use and rest our tongues in our mouths), and the spout held in the mouth over time may impact dentition, palate formation, and facial features. While research is needed to determine how long a child should use a spouted sippy cup, you may decide to limit them to occasional use over a few months. Or just skip them. With so many pop-up straw cups on the market that limit spills, it's possible!

SAFETY: A 2012 study by Nationwide Children's Hospital in Ohio reported that "a young child is rushed to a hospital every four hours in the U.S. due to an injury from a bottle, sippy cup or pacifier." As children are just learning to walk, they are often walking with a pacifier, bottle, or sippy cup in their mouths. One stumble and it can result in a serious injury. Kids need to be seated while eating and drinking. Limit pacifier use to bedtime after the age of 6 months and wean by 12 months. (Read more on pacifiers on page 93.)

360 Cups

In recent years, a spill-proof cup commonly referred to as "360" has been marketed to parents as a means to teach open-cup drinking while preventing spills. The name comes from the circular 360-degree top that allows a child to drink from any spot on the rim. The lid consists of a firm diaphragm that makes it spill proof. The problem with these cups is that they require the child to distort facial muscles and suck on the top to extract the drink. Speech pathologists prefer that parents don't use a 360 cup or limit them whenever possible. In order to drink from a 360, the child has to press down very firmly with the top lip, jut the jaw forward to brace against the cup, and distort the cheek and chin muscles to extract the liquid. This is not how children drink from an open cup and represents a different motor pattern than required for open or straw cups. As your child's face is developing in the first three years of life, overactivation of muscles can cause some muscles to become dominant over others.

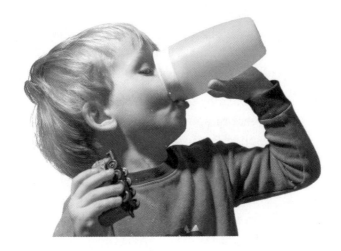

See how this little boy's cheeks suck in and the chin muscles have to over-activate to draw liquid from this cup? The lower lip and jaw juts forward because the top lip has to press down with force to expel the liquid.

Facial muscles for speech and feeding are intended to be balanced and work in harmony. It's best not to offer a cup that requires your child to drink in a peculiar fashion in order to stop spills.

If you've already purchased these cups, there are three solutions:

1. Some manufactures offer converter tops to turn the top into a standard lid with a straw. (See appendix, page 215.)

2. You may pop the top, exposing the rings of holes that allow the liquid to flow. Proceed with caution if you do so. Some children can manage the river of liquid, but others cannot. If the cup is filled to the top, the flow of the liquid will be minimal since it requires almost no tilting to pour into a child's mouth. But as the level of the liquid is reduced, the child must tilt the cup more (just like in an open cup) and there is no way to see how much liquid is about to cascade down the cup. Kids tend to tilt their head back when tilting a cup, especially when they cannot see what's inside. This opens up their airway, and kids who tilt their heads back are more at risk for aspiration. If you notice your child coughing

with this "topless" option, use the converter mentioned in #1 above.

3. Use the cup as a regular open cup with no lid at all.

How to Teach Straw Drinking

The prerequisite to learning to drink from a straw is being able to suck puree off a finger or a spoon. Most kids learn to do that within a week of starting solids. Because you'll want to teach this skill at 6 months, it's best to start with purees rather than water. The puree moves up the straw slower than a thin liquid like water and offers more control with less risk of taking a big suck and aspirating breast milk or formula before baby masters the skill. Most babies learn to drink from a straw in one day, if you break the lesson down into ten steps[11]:

1. Open a full jar of your child's favorite smooth, pureed baby food. Either homemade or store-bought is fine.

2. Dip a short, firm-sided straw in the puree, then let the tip fill about ½-inch full, so that there is puree inside and outside the straw. Put your finger on top of the straw to prevent the puree from spilling out the bottom.

3. With your finger still on the top of the straw, place about ½ inch of the wet straw flat on your child's tongue, as if it were a spoon of puree.

4. Wait for your child's lips to close around the puree on the tip, let go of the top hole, and slowly draw the straw straight out of their mouth. The tiny bit of puree that was on the outside of the straw is now on your child's tongue, ready to be swallowed.

5. Continue with this process until your child can manage a tiny bit more puree inside the straw. Remember, the outside of the straw should have a little puree on it, too, to tempt their lips to close around it.

6. Once your child has mastered steps 1 through 5 (this can take a few days of practice or happen all in one day), prime the straw with the puree 2 to 3 inches from the bottom by sucking on the top of the straw and then putting your finger over the top hole. Be sure to dip the bottom of the straw in just a tiny bit of puree, so that when you present it again, your child feels the puree on the outside.

7. To teach the next step, the suck, the key is to leave the straw in your child's mouth one or two seconds longer. Present the straw just as you would a spoon, wait for their lips to close . . . now wait again. As soon as they begin to suck, lift your finger off the top hole so that the puree can flow. Let your child suck slowly and swallow repeatedly until the straw is empty.

8. Once your child can manage two inches with ease, prime the straw to the top (four to five inches). Let your child practice sucking all the puree through the straw.

9. Take the full jar of food (or a covered cup filled to the top with puree) and leave about one inch of straw tip sticking out above the puree. Add a dab of puree to the tip of the straw again, just to encourage the sucking action. You may need to hold the jar or cup at a 45-degree angle so that the straw enters their mouth at just the right position while they learn to suck and prime the straw on their own.

10. Now that your child has mastered drinking purees via a straw, gradually thin the puree with water to nectar consistency and, eventually, to plain water. (Wait till baby is old enough to consume more water. For now, breast milk or formula can be enjoyed via a straw.)

Once your child can drink this way, it's time to cut the straw short enough that it extends just past the lips and barely touches the tip of the tongue resting in the mouth. Why? If the straw is too long, the tongue tip cannot lift to swallow properly.

Introducing the Open Cup

From the age of 6 months, parents can hold a tiny cup for baby to take small sips of water. Be sure baby is properly positioned in the feeding chair for learning this new skill. Limit baby to four to six ounces of water per day when drinking from a cup, as too much water is not good for babies and no baby should have plain water prior to 6 months of age because of risk of water intoxication. Until baby's motor control improves and they can pick up and control their own cup, you will need to hold the cup for them. Straw drinking is much quicker to learn, but both types of cups are introduced during the same month as solid foods. With close supervision, some ten-month-olds can drink from tiny cups independently, but they also love to dump and flood the table, too! Feeding therapists don't expect children to master independent cup drinking until 20 to 25 months of age. There's a tutorial to boost along this skill in your toddler in chapter four (page 145). A seven-month-old can easily manage their own straw cup if it is small enough and has a lid.

Right-Size Open and Straw Cups

For kids just starting out with a straw cup, choose one that has handles or is so small that their little fingers wrap securely around it. Ideally, the straw should be made of silicone to protect tender gums, but firm enough that they can't bite and flatten it. The width of the straw is also important. It should be as wide as a typical paper straw but narrower in the center due to the thickness of the silicone. The narrow channel in the middle prevents too much liquid from flowing into little mouths and delivers just enough for safe swallowing. The wider outer edge of the straw allows for lips to round and pucker, rather than kids biting or flattening their lips to take a drink. Rounding of the lips is the same movement kids use for many speech sounds, and drinking from the right straw helps to develop those muscles.

Straw cups sometimes contain valves to prevent the straw from leaking, but I'm not a fan of those cups. Most kids bite the straw and then sip, which is not a motor pattern that's helpful for feeding development. If the valve simply consists of a shelf of thin silicone near the very tip of the straw, I often cut the straw at the tip with sharp scissors and discard it. Other cups have the valve constructed just beneath the lid and it's sometimes possible to remove it altogether. Still, consider the length of the straw in your child's mouth. The tip of any straw should just reach the tip of the child's tongue resting behind their lower front teeth. Longer straws that reach over the tip of the tongue prevent the tongue tip from elevating to the alveolar ridge, just like a spouted sippy cup. For suggested cups, please refer to the appendix, page 215.

Pacifiers: Yay or Nay?

You might assume that because I want you to skip the sippy cup, I also want you to skip the pacifier. Not so! I recommend a specific type of pacifier for a short time for comfort and sleep. Providing baby with a pacifier while they are sleeping, even if the pacifier later falls from their mouth, has been found to reduce the risk of SIDS especially in the first six months of life. The AAP and the American Academy of Family Physicians recommend weaning kids from pacifiers between six and 12 months to prevent middle ear infections.[12] Because baby is using the forward-backward movement of the tongue to extract breast and bottle milk, the same movement on the pacifier is complementary to liquid feedings, although you may have decided to wait to offer a pacifier until breastfeeding is established in the first few weeks of life. Once solids are introduced, the more mature swallow pattern is essential for age-appropriate feeding development by 12 months, and maintaining pacifier use past this threshold may hinder baby's ability to learn to eat more advanced textures.

The shape of baby's pacifier is crucial. A popular pacifier used in many hospital nurseries is the Avent Soothie pacifier, which follows the AAP guidelines and is constructed of a single piece of pliable material for safety. Inspect any pacifiers frequently to ensure that no small pieces are becoming detached, especially if baby is teething. Features to shop for include pliable one-piece construction with no hard, plastic shields; ventilation holes to prevent moisture on the skin around the lips; and a long, cylindrical nipple. Flat or bulbous nipples and those promoted as "orthodontic" are strongly discouraged by most orofacial myologists (professionals, including speech pathologists, who have advanced training in facial development) due to concern that they may influence correct development of facial features.

How to Wean from the Pacifier

By 6 months, baby is ready to limit the pacifier to bedtime. Creating a routine to keep the pacifier in the bed will be comforting to baby and to you. Having weaned both of my children from their beloved "pacis," I can assure you that it's harder on the parent than the kid. You can do it in three simple steps:

1. **Create a paci-house.** A special box near the bed is where the pacifier will rest when not in use. When baby awakes, say, "Good morning, love! Pacifier goes in the paci-house." Hold the box open and let baby deposit the pacifier there. Immediately pick up baby and walk out of the room, leaving the box out of reach of little hands.

2. **As you put baby down to sleep, only provide the pacifier if baby requests it through vocalizations or gestures.** Out of sight, out of mind! Always include a transition object, like a blanket or baby-safe stuffed animal for baby to cuddle with during your bedtime routine, but do not put the object in the crib, per AAP recommendations. This object will provide comfort during waking hours instead of baby's relying on the pacifier.

3. **Between 6 and 8 months, consider complete weaning once baby has settled into this new bedtime routine.** If your child begins to suck fingers or thumb as a substitute, restore the paci and wait till the first birthday to wean. It's much harder

to wean from thumb sucking than from the pacifier, but by baby's first birthday it's time to eliminate the pacifier all together, and baby is less likely to adopt finger or thumb sucking as an alternative.

4. **Look under car seats, sofas, and throughout the house for any stray pacifiers!** The key to this method is to parent consistently, and if baby finds a random pacifier hiding under a chair, you'll have to start the process all over.

Weaning from the pacifier takes about three days. Pick a weekend when you'll have moral support from friends and family, and parent bravely.

Bottle Weaning

As described earlier in this chapter, baby will gradually begin to reduce the number of bottles per day once a feeding schedule has been established. (See chapter three, page 134, to learn how to eliminate the final bottles.) But if daytime bottles are still part of your child's routine, ask yourself the following questions:

- Is baby associating the bottle with a routine? Riding in the car seat, soothing before naptime, and reading books together are common scenarios. Provide alternatives, like a chewie, to occupy hands and mouth during story time.

- Is baby on a feeding schedule, allowing a bit of hunger to prompt the desire for solid foods? Or is baby drinking a bottle at a consistent time of the day that reduces the appetite for solid foods? Eliminate that bottle and keep baby occupied till it's time for the meal.

- Are you using the bottle for "ten minutes' peace?" You definitely deserve a break, but it's time to find a different form of self-care, because bottles aren't forever.

Common Early Challenges & How to Navigate Them

Being a responsive feeder includes learning how to navigate common behaviors like throwing food or tossing plates and utensils and deciphering why your child is so darn wiggly at the table! Throughout your child's lifetime, the best way to determine why your kids are behaving a certain way (good or bad!) is to consider these three things:

1. What cued the behavior

2. The behavior itself

3. What your child gets out of behaving that way

Behavior can be desired (good behavior) or undesired. Babies are busy discovering their world and become easily distracted by sounds and sights in their environment. The two of you may experience the occasional diversion when the dog runs into the room or if there are other kids laughing in another room. How then, do you know if that means your child has lost interest in eating? Here are three common challenges and how to navigate them in a responsive manner the first few times you observe your child throwing, tossing, or wiggling. By considering what cued the behavior and what happened afterward, you'll prevent these behaviors from becoming habits that interfere with your time at the table.

The Food Thrower

Young babies throw food because they have discovered gravity. It's fun! Luckily, there are plenty of other opportunities throughout the day to learn that same concept, and it's not necessary to reinforce it at mealtimes. When kids throw food or drop it on the floor, ignore it. Don't look down. Pretend you never saw it. As you continue to engage with baby, use your foot to slide the thrown food under the table or high chair. If you suspect that your little quarterback is tossing food for other reasons than for fun, consider these possibilities and how to respond.

Is baby overwhelmed by too much food?	Always offer a tablespoon or two of each food, possibly less for this baby. When baby would like more, offer more in very small portions.
Is baby signaling they are full?	Model the signs *all done* and *more*, in that order (see page 69). Babies will often imitate the last sign, so ask again. Now model *more* and *all done*, in that order. Remember to pause and give baby time to respond with their attempt to signal what they want. If they communicate "all done," remove baby lovingly from the high chair. Do not offer food again for older babies until the next scheduled eating time, once that schedule has been established.
Is baby frustrated by lack of skill?	Adapt the food to increase confidence. For example, if baby is tossing food because it's too slippery, cut it into an easier shape to grasp or coat it with bread crumbs.
Does baby just not like that food?	Ignore throwing and vary what is offered at that meal, including the suspected disliked food occasionally. If baby continues to toss that food, it's still important to offer it occasionally in the coming months. Young babies rarely toss foods that they don't like. They might remove it from their mouth or simply not pick it up at all. Older toddlers, who tend to be more opinionated about foods, won't learn to throw foods out of objection if you ignore it from the beginning. We'll explore this concept more in chapter three (page 129).

The Plate Tosser

Like food throwing, kids who toss their plates or simply tip them over do so for the sake of discovery and fun! Follow the same guidelines as above, but also consider using a plate or bowl that sticks well to the tabletop or tray. For suggested products, please refer to the appendix, page 215.

The Wiggler

Babies wiggle, twist, and turn for a variety of reasons. Although it may signal that they are done or not interested, it's often due to poor seating, soiled diapers, or other distractions. If you're seeing this behavior, consider the following questions and how to respond:

Is baby feeling stable and secure while seated?	Refer to the illustration on how to position your child in a high chair (page 50). Revisit the guidelines for positioning baby in their chair as they grow. Your high chair may need to be adjusted for changes in baby's height and weight each month.
Did baby soil their diaper?	In the first two years of life, the gastrocolic reflex activates as the belly begins to fill. It's quite common for babies to have a bowel movement in the middle of a meal. Toddlers gain better control of this urge when they begin potty training. Watch for tips on this in chapter five (page 132).
Is there a distraction that can be minimized?	Sensory distractions that may not be obvious to us can be very disruptive for babies. Look around the room and listen and watch baby for clues as to what is interrupting their ability to sit still. Is it the ceiling fan humming behind them or the feel of that new bib on their neck?
Is there an internal distraction?	Babies who wiggle, arch their backs, or move their bodies about with a look of discomfort on their faces may be struggling with gastroesophageal reflux, stomach pain due to constipation, or other medical issues. If the behavior continues, call your pediatrician.

The Overly Enthusiastic Eater

Some kids are just born with a passion for food! Parents often think kids eat so fast because they are so darn hungry! But that's rare, since most kids are on a meal and snack time schedule by their one-year birthday. Some kids just love the sensation of all the yumminess and haven't learned to pace themselves. However, their enthusiasm can lead to choking, so it's best to find creative ways to slow down the pace. Try the following tips to help:

1. Smaller pieces in tiny places. Whether baby is just developing the pincer grasp or has a more mature grasp, small pieces of food in individual compartments of an ice cube tray require a bit more time to pick up. It still takes time for younger babies who may feel frustrated with the tinier pieces when they are in separate compartments. Consider alternating the sizes to give baby practice with both.

2. Alternate offering small pieces and handheld solids on the plate, offering small sips of water occasionally to help wash away any remnants of food. Don't offer drinks when kids are stuffing—it's just too much to manage in a little mouth.

3. Encourage dipping. It's one more step before putting the food in the mouth, and it can add some moisture to help learning eaters chew and swallow more efficiently.

4. Place a few small pieces on one side of the high chair tray, encouraging baby to reach across midline (the center of their body) with the opposite hand to get it. Crossing midline is good for body and brain development, and it will slow down the eager eater.

5. Hold an espresso cup or small teacup and let them reach in to grab each piece of food. Serve a few pieces at a time this way to slow the pace and keep it fun!

The Stuffer

Got a little chipmunk at home? Why is it that some babies stuff those cheeks and then have trouble swallowing what they've pocketed in the gumlines? Are they even aware that food is stuck in those little cheeks? Many babies need a little wake-up brushing, helping to alert the inside of the mouth that it's time to pay attention. Once seated in their high chair, hand baby a double-sided toothbrush and show them how to brush inside the mouth, especially in those sweet cheeks. By alerting the nerve endings inside the mouth with gentle brushing, many kids become more aware of what's happening inside. Overstuffing can be due to poor oral awareness, and the brushing wakes up the mouth before parents offer food. Kids tend to stuff when the pieces are too big, too frequent, or presented way too fast.

After brushing, offer a preloaded fork intended for learning eaters. Show your child how to place small bits of food that have been pierced on the fork directly to the sides or lateral gums. Babies as young as 5 to 9 months will reflexively bite down on anything pressing on the gums beside the cheek. This placement ramps up the chewing motion. The smaller one-at-a-time offerings encourage swallowing. Watch for baby to swallow before handing them another forkful to place in their own mouth. If you're doing a hybrid approach of purees and baby-led weaning, it's fine to offer the fork to baby's mouth. Just wait to do so until you see that baby has swallowed most of the previous piece. Remember, keep the pieces small (about the size shown on the fork in the picture) and squishable for easy chewing. With this method, you're setting the pace, and it's not as easy to stuff. Just as for the child who eats too fast, dips will also help. The moister the food, the less likely it will lodge in those sweet cheeks.

Tips on Dips

Ranch dressing and ketchup are fine, but why not create your own flavorful and nutritious dips in just a matter of minutes? Try combining banana puree and nut or seed butter. Potato flakes, nutritional yeast, or infant cereal added to almost any pureed food makes a fabulous thickener, with added nutrition to boot! Blend ingredients from a main dish (e.g., chili or lentil stew) for a savory dip. Sweeter options include a beet blended with banana and yogurt. Almost anything can be turned into a nutritious dip!

Chapter Three

It's the Pace,
Not the Race

· 12 TO 18 MONTHS ·

Baby's first birthday marks the start of big transitions in development! Between the ages of 12 to 18 months, some feeding reflexes have integrated or faded into the nervous system. Over the next six months, you'll observe baby eating more solids instead of relying on breast milk or formula for the majority of nutrition. To match that keen interest in solid foods, new teeth are erupting. One of the biggest transitions is a child's newfound mobility: The first few steps somehow morphed almost overnight into walking and even running. You officially have a toddler in the house.

Shortly after baby's first birthday, you'll notice that many of the reflexes mentioned in chapter one seem to have disappeared. The integration of reflexes simply means that baby can now control these involuntary movements and has learned to do them on their own. However, there are two reflexes that should never integrate: the swallowing reflex and the gagging reflex.

The swallowing reflex is triggered hundreds of times each day without our even thinking about it. Yet, if I asked you to "swallow" you'd be able to do it intentionally because you understand the concept and the basic movements needed to elicit the swallow. In the next chapter, you'll learn how to use language and visuals to teach your baby to swallow with intention, but the reflex itself will still be present.

The gag reflex is also still present but activated farther back on the tongue and deeper in the mouth. Over the next several months you'll notice that baby gags less with food manipulated at the front and center of the mouth because the gag reflex has shifted to the back quarter of the tongue. The reflex is also triggered if food tickles the sensitive sides of the pharynx (where our tonsils are located). If you've ever had a throat culture at the doctor's office and gagged almost immediately, you know the feeling!

The bite reflex has integrated, no longer involuntarily activating the jaw muscles to bite down on spoons, fingers, or food. It has now completely shifted to biting and chewing soft foods with voluntary control, setting the stage for more advanced foods in the coming months. This repetitive motion of biting, chewing, and then swallowing is quite the workout for little mouths. Because of the gradual shift from breastfeeding or bottle-feeding to consuming more solid foods, baby has built up the stamina to eat more volume and a variety of safe textures. Babies who linger solely on purees past the ninth month of age become fatigued easily at mealtimes, due to their poor endurance for more advanced foods. Rotate purees throughout baby's diet, but make sure you're offering plenty of foods that require chewing to ensure proper mouth development.

Occasionally, you may notice **the tongue-protrusion reflex**, but it's less frequent by 13 months, at which time baby begins to favor a more mature swallowing pattern. By 18 months, it's very rare to see that same pattern in typically developing kids. Young toddlers who consistently use the less mature swallowing pattern of pushing the tongue forward with each swallow may need intervention by a pediatric feeding specialist. When toddlers try to progress to more challenging foods while stuck with an immature swallowing pattern, they can become picky eaters. Trying new foods that require chewing, placing the chewed food on the tongue, and then sending it back to be swallowed (when the immature pattern is to push it forward) is just too tricky! Kids quickly learn to limit their diets to just those foods they can swallow with ease, which are the same foods they ate in the first year of solids.

The transverse tongue reflex, which helps move the tongue from side to side, is still gradually integrating up to age two. When kids restrict the variety of textures and types of food they will eat, the learning curve for side-to-side movements suffers, too. Babies begin to gain control between the motor-window of 6 to 8 months. In the next phase of feeding, more foods are being offered that require slightly more advanced tongue movements. Toddlers are now relying on solid foods for the bulk of their nutrition and need the oral motor skills to bite, chew, and swallow a variety of healthy options.

Reliance on Fingers & Fists

Your one-year-old's little fingers have become precise at picking up small pieces of food, and your child is no longer raking with all four fingers to push pieces into the palm of their hand. This mature pincer grasp is now accurate and precise, forming the perfect OK symbol around each morsel and expertly placing it in the mouth. You'll also notice better control once the food is behind the lips, thanks to the transverse tongue reflex mentioned above. Toddlers now have a better awareness of their hands in space, even when they can't see their hands. Over the past several months, the repeated practice at self-feeding has assisted brain signals to interpret exactly where the food is and how to use the index finger to help move it about if needed. Little fists now grasp foods and utensils with ease, although the finesse of bringing a spoon up to the mouth without flipping it over and spilling down their front takes more time.

You Provide, Your Child Decides

"Variety is the spice of life" is true for toddler nutrition, too! The greater the variety of food groups offered to baby, the better likelihood that your little one is getting the best nutrition to grow and thrive. For children who need to be on specialized diets due to allergies, family food culture (e.g., vegetarian), or medical reasons, always consult with your pediatrician and a pediatric registered dietitian for specific guidelines for your family's needs.

Your toddler is now on a consistent schedule for meals and snacks, and most of their nutrition comes from solid foods. However, just like responsive breastfeeding and bottle feedings, try your best not to get too caught up in how much your child *should* be eating. Although I share suggested serving sizes throughout this book, they are guidelines. The ultimate expert on how much your child should be eating is your child—because they know when they feel full and when they are still hungry. No matter what age, there is one rule to remember when practicing responsive feeding: You provide, your child decides. It's your job to provide a variety of foods, and your child decides how much to eat.[1]

What Foods to Offer

Between 12 and 18 months, continue to offer safe, squishable solids and safely cut pieces of a wide variety of foods, as described on page 107. The difference now is that baby will eat more of it. It's the pace, not the race. Over the past six months, your little one has built endurance for maintaining a steady pace for biting, chewing, and swallowing without fatiguing before they are satisfied. It's the steady pace that's important, and there is no prize for kids who start eating more challenging foods or take bigger bites than their peers when it's not age appropriate from a developmental standpoint. Kids who appear to manage foods like big bites of bagels or who bite off the entire top of a broccoli spear are not advanced; they are just lucky. Keep a close eye on your child to ensure that they continue to take reasonably sized bites and remind others to offer only safe foods. Your child's airway is still narrow, and too large a bite or too advanced a texture may lead to a choking episode.

Knowing what foods to offer is easy, if you ask yourself these five questions:

1. Is it squishable?
2. Is it cut safely?
3. Am I offering most of the same ingredients that are on my own plate?
4. Am I offering mixed foods and single ingredients for variety (e.g., veggie lasagna or bits of taco meat with shredded cheese on the side)?
5. Am I rotating through foods for exposure to all kinds of flavors and safe textures?

Overreliance on Purees in Pouches

"Pouches of pureed fruits and vegetables have dominated growth in the baby-food aisle over the past decade," according to a 2019 article in the *Wall Street Journal*.[2] Those little packets of convenience seem to be every parent's dream, filled with all sorts of fruits and vegetables, sometimes with a little chia or quinoa mixed in. Kids push up the puree and suck it right down in a flash, and now little bellies and parents feel satisfied.

In an article for the American Speech-Language-Hearing Association, I expressed my concerns about the overreliance on pouches. Later, the *New York Times* article "Rethinking Baby Food Pouches"[3] shared my views. I'm not a big fan of those plastic bags of puree, but I'm not suggesting that you avoid them altogether. When parents and kids rely on pouches daily, it's just too much of what they perceive to be a good thing. Let's examine the pros and cons of feeding kids via daily pouches of puree and possible compromises so that we don't have to eliminate the convenience of pouches[4]:

Parents tell me that the convenience of pouches, with the knowledge that their children are consuming fruits and vegetables, is the number one reason they buy them. As a parent myself, I can understand that reasoning. The bigger issue is that kids benefit from being exposed to a variety of foods via food prep in the kitchen. Even toddlers can help wash and peel carrots using a kid's safety glove, snap green beans, and use kid-safe knives on softer fruits and cooked vegetables. The exposure to the textures and aromas, and being involved with parents in the kitchen, are what leads to kids' venturing to take a taste. A pouch on occasion for convenience is fine. Just don't let a pouch take the place of opportunities for food exploration.

The nutritional punch of whole fruits and veggies can't be beat, and most pouches don't compare to whole foods in terms of fiber content and overall nutrition. Check the ingredients to see how much fruit is in each one—most have applesauce as the first ingredient and contain up to 20 grams of natural sugar. That's a lot of sugar (even the natural kind) getting absorbed quickly into a small child's bloodstream.

While I'm a fan of purees and handheld foods, overreliance on purees via pouches can impede feeding development. Whenever possible, squirt the puree into a bowl and offer a spoon. Choose a savory pouch that isn't so high in sugar or puree flavorful leftovers ahead of time when meal prepping for the week.

Parents are often confused by the spout on the pouch, assuming that it's just like sucking from a straw. In fact, the spout does not require sucking at all, and for those children who do close and sip on the spout, the muscle action is so weak it doesn't provide the same benefit for facial development as straw drinking. Kids typically squeeze the pouch at the same time, squirting puree directly into the mouth with very little muscle engagement of the lips, jaw, and tongue.

Some children in feeding therapy or with special needs may start with pouches as a bridge to straw drinking and spoon feeding. But for typically developing kids, part of the allure is that pouches are quick to consume and less messy than other foods. When you're in a rush and need to eat on the go, a pouch on occasion is a nice solution. Just don't become dependent on them, and offer them only a few times a week at most. Chewing helps build the muscles children need for speech and feeding development and for appropriate facial and jaw growth. Squishing food from a pouch is fine for astronauts, but it should not be a daily method of eating for children.

Alternatives to Pouches

Purees from a store-bought pouch are expensive and not always the most nutritious. Make your own from bits of leftovers. A banana and half a baked sweet potato is a sweet and simple option. A beet from your salad, blended with some yogurt and a chunk of banana, is another easy choice. Offer it in a straw cup for the same convenience as a pouch without the added cost.

How Big Is a Portion?

I always suggest offering small samples of all the foods you'll be serving to your toddler. The simplest guideline is one tablespoon of each food multiplied by your child's age. So, for your one-year-old, start with one tablespoon of each food. As you get to know your child's appetite, you might decide to offer a bit more. We know that some children have keener appetites than others and by now, you are gauging your child's food responsiveness quite well.

Keeping portions small is helpful for three reasons:

1. It provides the opportunity for your child to decide and communicate if they'd like more.
2. It exposes your child to a variety of foods and doesn't emphasize favorites.
3. It reduces food waste.

How Big Is a Meal?

The number of food options is important, too. In general, limit the options to three or four foods per meal. Your one-year-old would start a meal with just one tablespoon each of four different foods on their plate. When your child requests more, you'll develop a sense of how much more to offer, but it likely will only be one or two tablespoons at a time. They can continue to have more servings throughout the meal, if it's prepared and available. To help you remember, think of M for meals, which means kids can have *more*. Snacks, however, are different.

How Big Is a Snack?

Snacks are just big enough for your child to hold in the palm of their hand. Some toddlers may need five mini meals per day rather than three larger meals and two small snacks. Certain medical conditions, like cystic fibrosis, type 1 diabetes, or metabolic disorders, often require larger snacks and mini meals. But in general, once a child reaches 18 months of age, the rule of thumb is to limit the size of snacks so that kids come to the table hungry (but not hangry) for breakfast, lunch, and dinner. In most cases, water is the ideal beverage to serve with a snack to ensure that kids don't fill up on milk or heavier liquids.

While M is for meals/more, think of S for small snacks. which means STOP. No seconds. Keep snacks small so that your child's hunger drive aligns with the family mealtime schedule and there is more opportunity for them to experience a variety of foods throughout the day. Because snacks are smaller than meals, the portion might include just one or two foods. Choose healthy options like a few whole wheat crackers smeared with peanut butter or a small dish of a delicious leftover. Prepackaged fish crackers are always fun, but snack foods don't have to come from the snack aisle at the grocery store. A nice soft piece of cheese and a few raspberries on the side are just as easy to offer and much more nutritious.

Put an End to Grazing

When kids want more snacks but you sense it's not in response to hunger, the best response is to reassure them that more food at a meal is coming soon. You can say, "That's what we have for snack right now. We will have lunch when we get back from the park." Grazing on snacks throughout the day throws off the feeding schedule and prevents your child from tuning in to their hunger and satiety cues. Grazing also changes the pH in the mouth, making it more acidic and leading to tooth decay. Unless there is a medical concern, kids who graze are eating for reasons other than a need for nourishment. They may become emotional eaters rather than mindful, intuitive eaters.

At times, it may seem confusing to follow a responsive feeding model and then not offer more food if your toddler appears hungry. Keep in mind that you have already begun to establish a hunger schedule at this point, and that you may need to adjust slightly depending on your child's unique appetite. It's a gradual shift over time, and you've been laying the foundation for a regular meal and snack time schedule for months. If your toddler has had a particularly active morning and you sense you should offer a bit bigger snack, you have that flexibility. The schedule is meant to guide you and prevent kids from grazing throughout the day. Watch their cues, know that appetites shift day to day in toddlers, and try your best to stick to a schedule while still reading your toddler's cues. Remember, it's a dance. The choreography is there to guide you, but if you'd like to add your own flair or a twirl or two because it suits your family's feeding style best, I support you.

How Many Veggies Do They Need?

Want to offer more veggies, but not sure how much is enough? Picture your toddler holding a chicken egg in each hand. The amount of vegetables that your child needs each day fits into each egg. Try serving some peas or corn kernels in a tiny cup for snack time, along with a bit of protein or fat. It doesn't need to be much, but it adds up throughout the day when all you need is two small eggs' worth of veggies.

Simple and Safe Shifts in Nutrition

Parents ask me a lot about nutrition! Although I need to know simple and safe facts about nutrition to support the families who consult with me as an SLP, the true experts in the field are pediatric registered dietitians (RDs). Always take counsel from a dietitian for specialized nutrition advice. Kacie Barnes of mamaknowsnutrition .com is a Registered Dietitian Nutritionist (RDN) with a keen interest in baby and toddler nutrition. I consulted with Kacie to ensure that the guidelines suggested in the following are ideal for toddlers from 12 to 36 months:

ADVICE FROM AN EXPERT REGISTERED DIETITIAN NUTRITIONIST

CARBOHYDRATES

Who doesn't love carbs? Kids seem to crave them, and the most hesitant eaters I work with limit their diets to crunchy fish crackers, noodles, fries, and breaded chicken nuggets. In fact, carbohydrates should be about 50 percent of your toddler's diet, because they are their main source of energy. However, there are two types of carbs, simple and complex, and it's the latter that are the richest in fiber, vitamins, and the nutrition to help kids feel energized throughout the day. Complex carbohydrates include vegetables, whole grains, beans, and lentils, and it's these energy boosters and brain builders that should be most plentiful on your child's plate. Simple carbohydrates can be natural, whole foods, like fruit. For example, a few (safely cut) apple sticks can supply that quick burst of fuel at snack time to help kids maintain their energy till the next meal, especially if combined with a bit of protein, like a schmear of thinned almond butter for dipping. But simple carbs can also be processed or "refined," and those tend to be quick and easier to grab on the go.

While they may be convenient, snacky foods like fish crackers, containers of dry cereal, or some packaged snack bars may include white flour and sweeteners that create a quick lift in energy, followed by a crash in insulin and a cranky kid! It's the roller-coaster ride of simple carbs that causes children to want to graze throughout the day, complaining of hunger shortly after that snack and reaching once again for that same food without ever feeling truly satisfied. A bit of those foods is fine, but there are three rules for ensuring sound nutrition for your child: Offer variety, variety, and more variety.

PROTEIN

Parents seem to worry about how much protein their kids need, but surprisingly, kids don't need as much as you might think. In fact, now that your toddler has turned one, 13 grams of protein—about the equivalent of one egg and a cup of whole milk—will do the trick! According to Barnes, other terrific sources of protein include meats, tofu, beans, cottage cheese, low-sugar yogurts, and hemp seeds. Make sure to expand beyond dairy protein sources. While milk, cheese, and yogurt are often favorites for toddlers, they won't contribute the iron your child needs. Meat and fish are the best protein sources of iron, but iron can also be found in vegetarian protein sources like beans, lentils, and tofu.

FAT

Babies and toddlers need healthy fats to support body and brain growth. They also metabolize fats, an important energy source, at a more rapid rate than adults. Fats help your child absorb other nutrients essential for growth and development, but not every fat is beneficial to growing bodies. Barnes recommends that parents strive to offer foods that contain monounsaturated and polyunsaturated fats, limit saturated fats, and avoid trans fats.

- Monounsaturated fats include olive, safflower, and canola oils. Avocados and nuts (remember to chop them into baby-safe pieces) are healthy options, too.

- Polyunsaturated fats provide two important fatty acids: omega-3 (found in formula and breast milk) and omega-6. Both are important for children's brain and body health. However, for those families that consume liberal amounts of processed food, the higher amounts of omega-6 can lead to behavioral and learning issues in children. A balance of omega-3 fats may help manage these conditions. Common sources of whole foods containing omega-6 fats include nut butters, eggs, and corn oil. Omega-6 is plentiful in most diets in general, but omega-3s are not, especially after the first year of life. To ensure that toddlers have adequate sources, offer plenty of salmon, sardines, and low-mercury fish. Ground flaxseeds or whole chia seeds are an excellent source and easily added to muffins, pasta sauce, and even breaded chicken fingers! Omega-3 fats are essential for healthy development of the central nervous system, cardiovascular system, and lifelong eye health. Children one to three years of age need 0.7 grams of omega-3 fat per day.[5]

- Saturated and Trans Fats: Saturated fats can support growth and development, if offered wisely and not in excess. Natural sources include meat and dairy products. Trans fats are found in processed foods, such as some snack foods, cookies and cakes, and fried foods. Watch for terms like "hydrogenated" or "partially hydrogenated" oils on an ingredient list. Those terms refer to trans fats, which have no health benefits for children or adults. Like saturated fats, trans fats can raise cholesterol and increase the chance of getting heart disease, with risk building over time. It's best to avoid trans fats and be conscious of limiting saturated fats found in foods such as butter, stick margarine, red meat, and processed meats.[6]

FIBER

If your toddler is getting a variety of foods each day, it's likely there's enough fiber in their diet to reduce the chance of constipation. There's one thing I know for sure after twenty years of helping the pickiest eaters. Once a child becomes constipated, they are likely to be more hesitant about eating or trying new foods, because constipation causes a drop in appetite. Too much fiber may lead to the opposite dilemma: runny stools and diarrhea, including stomach cramping and discomfort when trying to eat. Both are common, but there are some easy guidelines to help your toddler feel comfortable while maintaining healthy bowel function.

The key is to offer both types of fiber, soluble and insoluble. Soluble fiber is found in many fresh fruits, oats, lentils, beans, chia seeds, and vegetables like peas and carrots. Its main job is softening the stool to aid in having a daily bowel movement (BM) but soluble fiber can also help regulate blood sugar levels. Insoluble fiber is found in whole wheat flour, bran, nuts, and vegetables like cauliflower, green beans, and potatoes. Its job is to absorb liquid and add bulk to the stool, which stimulates the urge to have a BM. Regular BMs no less than once every 2 or 3 days not only help a child feel most comfortable and eager to fill their belly with a variety of healthy foods but also support potty training, when the time comes. (Some children may need to have daily bowel movements to reduce symptoms of other medical issues, such as GERD, or to support appetite regulation for extreme picky eaters. See the section on constipation and appetite (page 121) for more information. Please refer to chapter seven to learn about red flags that indicate a need for a feeding evaluation for our more hesitant eaters (page 167).

Offering variety is key, but if you're a numbers person, Barnes explains that a one-year-old needs about 19 grams of fiber per day.[7] Limit refined white foods, avoid more than 2 or 3 servings of dairy daily, and encourage lots of exercise to help with regularity. Toddlers can now have free access to water, too!

WATER, MILK, JUICE, AND SUGARY BEVERAGES

There's a simple formula to ensure that your child is drinking enough water every day: Children's Hospital of Orange County recommends that kids ages one to eight drink an eight-ounce cup of water one times their age throughout the day (sipping, not guzzling!).[8] For toddlers, that would be as follows:

- One-year-old = 1 x 8 ounces of water per day
- Two-year-old = 2 x 8 ounces of water per day (and up to 34 ounces per day)[9]
- Three-year-old = 3 x 8 ounces of water per day (and up to 40 ounces per day)[10]

Multiple studies indicate that when kids drink adequate amounts of water and remain hydrated throughout the day, they can pay better attention, learn well, and become less fatigued compared to peers who were even mildly underhydrated.[11] Fostering a love for water in toddlers leads to a lifelong healthy habit! Learn more about fun ways to serve water and encourage kids to help themselves in an upcoming chapter.

A good sign of hydration is pale yellow urine in the toilet, or several wet diapers throughout the day. Clear urine is not necessary, so do not worry that your child is underhydrated if you see a yellow tint.

Your one-year-old can now drink whole milk. Prior to this transition, you offered cheese and other dairy products to baby, but drinking milk had not yet been an option. If baby has tolerated other dairy products well, begin offering whole milk now till age two. Kids older than two may be transitioned to lower-fat milk (skim or 1%) if their pediatrician has no concerns about their growth trajectory. Dairy milks provide calcium, vitamin D, protein, and other essential nutrients, but according to Barnes, soy milk can, too. According to the AAP, "soy milk is nutritionally equivalent to cow's milk and is an acceptable alternative" for kids with dairy intolerances or when a family's food culture does not include cow's milk. Plant-based milks (almond, pea, and so on) often contain added sugars and are not as dense in terms of nutrients. Be sure to consult with an RD if your child requires a special diet that includes these possible alternatives.

The AAP discourages parents from serving toddler formulas. "Often marketed by formula companies as 'transitional' to wean from breast milk or formula, [toddler milks] are unnecessary and potentially harmful to young children. These products contain added sugars and may fill a baby's stomach up so he or she is not hungry for healthier foods."[12]

Kids under the age of one should only be served juice for medicinal purposes, such as to relieve constipation. In the transition phase of age one to three, kids can have 100 percent fruit juice (with no sugar added) if limited to just 4 ounces per day.[13] Consider diluting the juice with water and offering it only on occasion, rather than daily. Blending a whole orange with all the pulp or an apple with the skin, then diluting with water or freezing into an ice pop is a delicious twist that will include the phytonutrients and fiber missing from most strained, store-bought juices.

Beverages with added sugars include flavored milks, soda pop, sports drinks, lemonade, and some sparkling waters. Avoid sugary drinks, as they increase your child's risk of childhood obesity, cavities, fatty liver disease, and other medical challenges like diabetes and heart disease. Please avoid artificial sweeteners unless they are needed to make a specialized diet for a medical condition more palatable. We will go deeper into the pros and cons of restricting sugar and other sweet foods in older children in chapter five (page 170).

Sodas, sports drinks, and whipped icy drinks from the local coffee shop contain both added sugars and caffeine. Young children should never consume caffeinated beverages, as these leads to irritability, difficulty concentrating, agitation, headaches, gastroesophageal reflux, heart palpitations, and hyperactivity.

CALCIUM, VITAMIN D, AND IRON

Toddlers from ages one to three need 500 mg of calcium per day, which can come from a variety of sources. If baby is still breastfeeding, breast milk will contribute calcium—an essential mineral for building strong bones and teeth and for optimal muscle functioning. Other good sources include cheese, yogurts, fortified soy products, whole milk, fortified breads and cereals, oranges, broccoli, peas, beans, and hearty leafy greens like kale or collard greens.

Optimal calcium absorption is dependent on vitamin D, Barnes explains. Alarmingly, your child's bone density and bone strength can be reduced due inadequate levels of this powerhouse vitamin. Toddlers need 600 IU (international units) per day. I'll never forget a precious two-year-old whose caring parents came to me asking for help with his extremely picky eating habits. Just prior to my assessment, he had begun to limp and walk with an unsteady gait, and after months of detective work and suspicions of a neurological disorder, doctors finally diagnosed him with rickets due to severe vitamin D deficiency. While nutritional rickets is rare in children, studies indicate that incidents have dramatically increased in the last twenty years.[14] Yet vitamin D deficiencies are common for several reasons. First, parents have been diligent about protecting kids from the rays of the sun. Second, pediatric feeding disorders (PFDs), which may impact children nutritionally, occur in 1 out of 4 typically developing kids. Third, poor absorption can also be the culprit. Fourth, even when parents offer a variety of foods, there just aren't many foods that contain this powerhouse vitamin. Eggs have small amounts (20 IU per egg), and fortified milk will also contribute some (about 100 IU per 8 ounces). Fatty fish like salmon and sardines are terrific sources, but the Food and Drug Administration (FDA) strongly recommends limiting consumption of fatty fish to just 3 to 4 ounces per week in young children.[15] Although I encourage you to limit juice, when you do choose to offer juice to your child, fortified orange juice is a terrific source of vitamin D. Pair foods containing vitamin D with higher-fat foods, such as an avocado, to increase absorption. Talk to your child's physician about how to limit sunlight exposure yet still benefit from brief exposure to daily sunlight in a safe manner (e.g., morning sun exposure is less intense than midday) and whether a supplement is appropriate for your toddler. Low levels of vitamin D have also been associated with a compromised immune system, severe asthma, and poor sleep in children.[16]

Kids who feel sluggish and tired may also be iron deficient. As discussed in chapter one (page 8), infants who are breastfed require iron drops as a supplement, but by 12 months of age toddlers who are eating a variety of foods may no longer need supplementation. Consult with your pediatrician to decide what's best for your little one. Iron deficiency is the most common cause of anemia, evidenced by a significant decline in red blood cells.

Signs of anemia in children may include pale skin, cheeks, or lips; irritability; fatigue; slow cognitive development, and difficulty maintaining body temperature. For more severe cases, your child may present with shortness of breath, dizziness or fainting, hair loss, and restless leg syndrome. Children may also be observed eating or craving unusual nonfood items such as crayons, paper, dirt, or ice. "Pica" is the term used for this behavior, and it will usually diminish once iron stores are reestablished, or kids may need a short period of feeding therapy to fade the habit.

Iron is plentiful in iron-fortified grains and cereals, red meat, and poultry (like duck or dark-meat chicken), egg yolks, beans, oatmeal, and some green vegetables (like spinach, kale, swiss chard, or beet greens). The key is to pair the iron-rich foods with other foods rich in vitamin C to enhance absorption, like tomatoes, oranges, or broccoli.

If you'd like to learn more about vitamins, minerals, and specific advice on childhood nutrition, refer to the appendix, page 215, for websites that I find most helpful, including Kacie's at mamaknowsnutrition .com.

Transitions in Appetite

By the end of the first year, your baby likely tripled their birth weight! The metamorphosis from infancy to an upright toddler, cruising the furniture and perhaps taking first steps, is astounding! As kids transition into their second year of life, Mother Nature pumps the brakes, and that rapid growth you witnessed in baby's first year begins to slow down. According to registered dietitian-nutritionists Jill Castle and Maryanne Jacobson, "Weight increases in the first year by 200 percent, body length by 54 percent, and head circumference by 40 percent, changes that are reflected in the hearty appetite of most babies."

In fact, the baby and toddler growth charts used by your pediatrician and developed by the World Health Organization (WHO) are designed to reflect the typical growth curves seen universally in young children. If every parent expected their baby's appetite and growth to be equivalent to that first year, imagine the difficulty we would have believing in responsive feeding and in our baby. One mom once said to me, teary eyed and worried about her fifteen-month-old, "But I've got to feed him more, he's barely grown at all compared to last year!" When we plotted baby's growth, she took a big sigh of relief when she saw the steady curve that illustrates how babies grow and thrive with the right nutrition. Trusting baby's communication and your ability to respond appropriately, rather than coaxing in "one more bite for Mommy" to ease your anxiety, is sometimes easier said than done. But you've been practicing responsive feeding techniques for six months, and baby grew superbly! Your toddler will, too, just at a different rate, because that's how nature intends kids to grow.

It's helpful to keep in mind that toddlers tend to eat less on some days and much more on other days. Don't assume the heartier appetite is only because of what was on the menu on that particular day. Keep rotating a variety of foods and do your best not to offer presumed favorites every day. Kids become adventurous eaters because they take tastes of a variety of foods over the course of a few weeks. This steady stream of taste testing builds the foundation for healthy eating for a lifetime.

Growth and Appetite

Appetite in toddlers seems to wax and wane, but growth should remain steady. Your child's doctor will plot their growth on a chart at each well-child visit or if you have concerns about your child's nutritional health. Just like adults, kids come in all shapes and sizes, and the growth curve is one tool to monitor your child's health, but it is not a) a competition, or b) a passing or failing grade. Growth charts compare populations (kids of the same sex and age) to provide the physician a visual of continuous growth or to detect if growth stalls. There will always be kids in the 1st percentile and others in the 99th percentile and plenty of kids in between. Steady, continuous growth is key, but it may not tell the entire story.

Pediatrician Dr. Nimali Fernando explained to me that a percentile on a growth chart is just a snapshot in time that tells us how a child compares to their age-matched peers in terms of weight and height. A growth *curve*, however, helps us know where a child has been and where they are now. It tells a story about a child's genetics, their nutrition, and their overall health. It's important to understand that a child's growth curve is just one piece of information and may not accurately give an overall picture without other key data. For instance, growth curves may not reflect the quality of the nutrition a child is getting, as is demonstrated by the fact that many obese kids are undernourished.[17]

Constipation and Appetite

Have you ever used a stool chart to monitor your child's bowel movements? Sounds a bit neurotic, right? Here's why I recommend it, for just a short time: It's very common to miss signs of constipation until your toddler's gut becomes uncomfortable and BMs are painful. Constipation is either a decreased frequency or the painful passage of a BM. According to the North American Society for Pediatric Gastroenterology, Hepatology, and Nutrition, "Children one to four years of age typically have a bowel movement one to four times a day. If not daily, more than 90% of children go at least every other day, although these children may be constipated."[18]

Monitoring a child's bathroom habits for a short period of time can reveal unexpected signs of constipation, including loose, liquid stools, which are the body's way of trying to clean out larger, impacted, solid stools from the intestines. Small pieces of stool resembling rabbit pellets may also signal that your child is constipated. For more signs of constipation, visit the "Constipation" page on gikids.org or the GI Kids channel on YouTube and watch the video "The Poo in You" to learn why it's important for kids to have regular, daily BMs. Google "Bristol Stool Chart" for a pictorial of what healthy, comfortable BMs look like—you might be surprised!

Short bouts of constipation impact a child's willingness to try new foods because a constipated child is not a hungry child. Hunger truly is the secret sauce when it comes to being an adventurous eater. Long-term constipation has also been shown to have a negative effect on growth in young children.[19] Now that your child has made the transition to more solid foods, remember to include water and a balance of soluble and insoluble fiber in their diet, along with plenty of exercise to facilitate regularity and gastrointestinal comfort.

Teething and Appetite

Several studies[20] have shown that children who are teething often suffer from decreased appetite, but any exhausted parent of a teething toddler could tell us that! The real question is, what do we do about it?

- Do gently rub your child's gums with a clean finger or "baby" washcloth moistened with chilled water.

- Do offer teething toys, making sure they are cleaned with soap and water regularly. Choose silicone, slightly flexible options.

- Do try an over-the-counter remedy recommended by your pediatrician. If your child is especially uncomfortable and can't seem to get relief, ask your child's doctor if you can use an over-the-counter pain remedy such as acetaminophen (e.g., Tylenol) or ibuprofen (e.g., Advil, Motrin).

- Do offer chilled or partially frozen and safely cut foods. Options for toddlers include partially thawed and halved blueberries or other pieces of fruit. Frozen veggies like corn, peas, and chopped green beans that have been thawed enough to squish between sore gums are terrific options, too! The smaller pieces work best, as longer strips in tiny hands can be too cold to hold.

- Do offer homemade ice pops cradled in a silicone ice pop holder. Milk products mixed with puree work best because they don't freeze into an extremely hard ice cube like water does. Ice cubes held on sore gums run the risk of injuring the gums if left there too long.

- Do offer small dots of frozen yogurt. Simply dot yogurt on a sheet of waxed paper resting in a shallow, covered container. Store the container in the freezer.

- Do offer silicone feeders filled with frozen fruit.

- Don't offer silicone feeders filled with water. Any ice cube held on a sore gum for long is too cold, and injury to gum tissue could result.

- Don't use teething rings filled with liquid or gel. They can break easily, and your child could ingest the contents.

- Don't use numbing gels, sprays, or other products containing benzocaine on children under the age of two. The Food and Drug Administration (FDA) states: "These products carry serious risks and provide little to no benefits for treating oral pain, including sore gums in infants due to teething."[21] Examples of common over-the-counter products that contain benzocaine include the brands Anbesol, Orajel, Baby Orajel, and Orabase.

- Don't use homeopathic teething tablets. The Mayo Clinic states: "In recent years, lab analysis of some homeopathic remedies found greater amounts than labeled of the ingredient belladonna, which can cause seizures and difficulty breathing."[22]

- Don't use baby or adult jewelry marketed for relieving teething pain. Sadly, children have choked on and been strangled by these products.[23] Concerns include potential injury to the mouth from infection. Just because something is marketed as a teether doesn't always mean it's safe.

Brush that Tongue

When brushing baby's gums and teeth, brush their tongue, too! It's important not only for oral health but also for feeding development. Brushing the tongue helps your child learn to tolerate new sensations, which in turn helps manage new food textures. It activates tongue movement, especially the lateral movements, for learning to chew and swallow safely. It also aids in shifting the gag reflex posteriorly to coincide with stages of feeding development.

Exercise and Appetite

Toddlers are busy. Every day brings a new life experience, from discovering how to blow bubbles in milk to encountering a caterpillar in the backyard. Activity builds appetite, and keeping kids on a feeding schedule will increase the likelihood that kids will try new foods. However, at this age, kids' attention span at mealtime can be fleeting. Transitions are also hard for toddlers, but there are several strategies that support responsive feeding and that will make the transitioning to and from the table much easier for everyone:

4. **Heads up for cleanup!** Young toddlers love to help with a brief tidying of the playroom when it includes a tidy-up tune. One minute of picking up toys while singing the cleanup song signals that toy-time is over and the next activity is about to begin. Having your child hold the basket while you gather up the toys is enough participation to aid them in moving to the next room for lunch. As discussed in chapter one, you're creating a loving routine in a predictable environment. This routine also supports shifting to the new environment in a smooth and predictable manner.

5. **Mark the beginning of the meal.** It's a special time! When kids engage in a foreseeable start to the meal, they transition much more easily than just putting them in their highchair.

Sing a mealtime song, say a prayer (it's so adorable when toddlers bow their little heads), or find a custom that suits your family's food culture. As discussed in the next chapter, older toddlers can hold your wrist while you light a candle in the center of the table. No matter what the custom, it's clear to everyone that the meal is about to start.

Thanks to the consistent and expected routines you've established, your child will likely communicate hunger and, naturally, you'll provide the meal. Parenting consistently helps your child predict what will happen, and that's comforting for any kid.

Your child experiences predictable, positive responses from you, reinforcing their attempts at communication. That's responsive feeding!

Utensils and Appetite

At about one year of age, many kids have mastered using a spoon independently. But for those who are still having trouble, a voracious appetite may be a factor. When kids are really hungry, utensils often get set aside, and kids just dig in with their fingers. It's much more efficient that way! Still, learning to use utensils is important, too. Set kids up for success with the following tips to master independent use of both a spoon and a child-safe fork:

Spoon or Fork: Which Comes First?

Typically, children make the best progress with utensils when a spoon is introduced first. But for older toddlers who are not progressing with utensil use, you may find that mastering the fork is easier for several reasons:

1. Once the food is pierced, it stays on the fork better than on a spoon.

2. Learning to use a spoon starts with a dip-and-flip motion. When kids are just learning to use a fork, they often use the

same motion, flipping the fork upside down to place it in their mouth. The two utensils support the same motor pattern.

3. Forks are just interesting! Some kids are fascinated by how they work but may easily get frustrated if they have difficulty piercing the food.

Start with one or the other at this age, rather than offering both at one meal. If your child is having trouble refining motor skills needed for utensil use, keep it simple. Offer a spoon for a few days and then switch to the fork, or vice versa. Once they appear more comfortable handling one or the other, you can begin to offer both at each meal. If your toddler begins to show a strong preference for one utensil over the other, return to the routine of offering just one at a time to ensure that they get the practice they need to boost their skills over time.

Boosting Self-Feeding Skills with Spoons

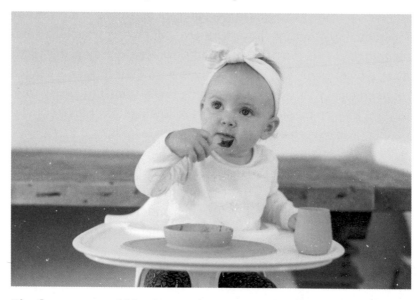

The first step to self-feeding with a spoon is the dip and flip, covered in chapter two. The next step requires a bit more control of the wrist motion and is best described as a dip, scoop, and turn of the wrist. It takes some time and coordination to combine all three motions into a smooth arc that delivers yummy food to their little mouths! Keep in mind that over time the movements will become more refined and that wrist and forearm rotation and finger movements will gain more precision and a higher quality of movement throughout the toddler years. If your toddler is having trouble mastering the three different movements, break it down into these three steps and gently encourage your child to build the fine-motor skill to self-feed.

1. The Dip and Flip: When starting self-feeding, most babies learn to dip between 6 and 9 months, just by watching a grown-up dip, too. They dip and flip the spoon over before bringing it up to their mouth.

2. The Dip, Scoop, and Flip: The scooping motion emerges between 9 and 11 months, and some babies will flip the spoon over before placing it in the mouth. You can help your child learn the very important "scoop" by pouring a thin line of yogurt across the bottom of a stay-put bowl for baby to follow before gliding it back up to eat.

3. The Dip, Scoop, and Turn: At about 14 to 18 months, after the scoop, kids learn to turn the wrist to bring food to their mouths rather than flipping the spoon upside down. This is where the older toddler may have some difficulty. Placing a large mirror on the table in front of their food (and out of reach) helps kids see the process in action. Modeling the three steps in slow motion can also be beneficial. Using gentle and encouraging hand-over-hand guidance with a favorite food aids the learning process, too. Outside of mealtimes, leave child-safe spoons in the sandbox or a sensory bin filled with clean, uncooked rice for kids to dip, scoop, turn, and dump into taller containers. Position the containers close to their bellies in the sandbox to mimic the motor pattern needed for self-feeding. Just watch them closely. Your toddler won't be the first to try a bite of sand!

Boosting Self-Feeding Skills with Forks

No matter how old a child is, learning to use a fork starts with four easy steps. With consistent practice, kids gain more finesse over time.

1. Offer safe, squishable pieces of food in a stay-put bowl that grips the table or high chair tray, so that the bowl won't move when kids press into it with the fork. The squish factor makes piercing with a fork much easier and is best for safer chewing and swallowing. Cubes of avocado, bananas, or steamed squash are all great choices. Silicone ice cube trays with cubes of food in each compartment are helpful, too, since each section creates a boundary for the fork to do the job. You'll need to steady the tray for your child while they are still learning how hard to pierce.

2. Show your child how to hold the table or the side of the bowl with the "forkless" hand. When kids stabilize with one hand, the other hand with the fork will gain better control.

3. Place the cubes in the left corners of the bowl if your child is holding the fork in their right hand and vice versa. Now they can poke down and brace the fork against the tall sides of the partitioned bowl.

4. Offer a fork that has a short handle and wide tongs to hold safe-size pieces. For my preferred products with these features, please refer to the appendix, page 215.

Which hand is the correct hand for toddlers to use?

Now is not the time for kids to develop a hand preference. Learning to use either hand means your child is also using *both* sides of their brain. You're working on your child's brain development (rather than developing hand dominance, typically seen closer to age three or even four) so parent proactively and encourage kids to learn to fork with both hands.

Common Responsive Feeding Scenarios & Types of Eaters

In chapter two, I explained that being a responsive feeder includes learning how to navigate common behaviors like throwing food, tossing plates and utensils, or deciphering why your child is so darn wiggly at the table! Throughout your child's lifetime, the best way to determine why they are behaving a certain way (good or bad!) is to consider three things:

1. What cued the behavior

2. The behavior itself

3. What your child gets out of behaving that way

These same principles hold true for the rest of your child's life, but especially in the toddler years, when your child's behavior may feel unpredictable and confusing to you.

Attention Is Your Child's Paycheck

Be incredibly careful what behavior you pay your child for. Be aware of those behaviors that you want to foster, and ignore behaviors that are undesired. It's not that you're ignoring your child, you are simply not paying attention to any behavior that gets in the way of good behavior. For example, throwing cups on the floor gets in the way of drinking milk. Ignore that. When kids are drinking their milk because they have a desire for it, give them attention by talking about cows and milk, or using words like "Brrrrr! Chilly milk in that cup!" When we engage immediately after the behavior, we are increasing the likelihood that the behavior will occur again.

The Learning Eater

Think of a toddler's first experiences with new solids like a classroom. Although you're in the class, too, consider yourself the teacher's aide. There are eight teachers leading the lesson, and they are your child's eight senses. Learning to eat is a sensory experience, and it takes time to interpret thousands of pieces of information about all kinds of new foods over the next several years. Your learning eater will want to smash blueberries one day to focus on the tactile and auditory experience (hear the *squoosh!*) and on other days eat so many blueberries that you'll be convinced those little blue fingertips will be stained forever. That's how all children learn, by stopping, pausing, and processing bits of information and then surging on full speed ahead! Because you are a responsive feeder, you'll observe and identify what sensory aspects are most appealing to your child and support them in the process. You're the aide. Your job is to support. Remember: The sensory system is the teacher.

The Food Explorer

What happens when your learning eater seems to be mesmerized by food play and exploration? It may be adorable when a toddler smashes avocado onto a spoon and insists on feeding the grown-up (but not themselves) or drums pieces of steamed carrots on the table like a budding rock star, but when is that kid going to actually eat? Between 14 and 18 months of age, children are entering a salient cognitive stage of pre-symbolic play, typically using familiar tools like utensils for pretend play based on everyday activities, like feeding Mommy. Between 19 and 22 months, you'll see the same type of play expand to two actions in row (e.g., toddler feeds a doll with the spoon and then does the same for Mommy). Kids are supposed to do this—their brain is telling them to explore and learn. Consequently, with mealtimes being three times a day (plus snacks), you're likely to observe long periods of food exploration from both a sensory perspective and a cognitive/play perspective. Combine that with a shift in appetite as compared to the first year of life, and it can feel like your toddler is never going to stop exploring and just eat. If it feels like too much play is getting in the way of eating, respond by not responding. Don't give the play any attention. Kids tend to play more when we engage with them. There are appropriate times to encourage and participate in food exploration, but it doesn't need to be at every meal if your child can't seem to move on to filling their belly. Remember, feeding responsively is a dance—and you don't always have to hop onto the dance floor. It's OK to sit this one out, for now.

The Cruiser

Toddlers are the busiest little creatures! There is so much of the world to explore, especially when just learning to cruise furniture, walk, and even run! Shortly after 18 months of age, with your help, toddlers can learn to take their plate to the counter to signal that they are all done. Watch for more on that strategy in the next chapter. For younger toddlers who want to get down from their highchair minutes after starting a meal, refer to the chart in chapter two regarding kids who wiggle and seem distracted in their high chair (page 98). Your toddler is likely wanting to get down for the same reasons, but now they are more mobile!

The Mess Maker

Feeding specialists encourage parents to let kids get messy. That's because sensory exploration is important for all stages of development. But, as a mom myself, I understand that sometimes, especially for toddlers, being a mess maker is way more fun than eating! When you feel that your child's interest in making a mess has taken the place of eating, or is just getting out of control, consider the following questions and responses.

Is your toddler getting too much attention for making a mess?	Attention is your child's paycheck. Even when a parent responds to spilt milk or an overly enthusiastic moment of sensory play with a "Hey, we don't throw food!" it's still attention. Instead, try to remove attention for behaviors that you'd like to fade away. A gentle reminder of what they can do instead is helpful, such as "Food stays here on your plate."
Is your toddler simply not that hungry?	Growth slows down significantly after the first year, and so does appetite. Rather than staying in the feeding chair and making too big a mess, it's OK to respond with "We're making a big mess. That tells Mommy you'd want to be all done. Show me 'all done' when you want to get down." For kids who can't yet sign or say "done," read their facial expressions and body language and respond with, "I can see you're all done. I'll help you get down."
Is there a way to minimize the mess?	Try an allover bib noted in the appendix. Some days we just need something to minimize the mess and let the kids keep exploring!

The Pooper

Have you noticed that when your child is in the midst of eating a meal, they often soil their diaper? It can be frustrating to stop in the middle of a meal to take a toddler to be changed. Still, it's part of how their little bodies work, thanks to a reflex we all have called the gastrocolic reflex. As we grow, we learn to regulate our bodies, and although the reflex is still ready when we need it, it no longer activates every time we eat.

As children approach age three, the urge will diminish, but they may occasionally need to be excused from the table to visit the bathroom. Always allow them to go, or constipation may result. But if your child is managing regular bowel movements at the same time most days, try not to give the actual "bathroom time" much attention while they are on the potty. Help them get cleaned up without any fanfare and head right back to the table. Avoid letting bathroom time be more fun than eating time or a way to get down and play.

The Chipmunk

In chapter two, I provided strategies for babies who tend to stuff their little cheeks and are overenthusiastic eaters. As kids learn to try new handheld foods such as small sandwiches, they can still stuff too much into their mouths, resulting in chipmunk cheeks packed with food. That makes it difficult to swallow safely. Refer to page 100 to review those tips and try the following strategy now that your toddler is older and can follow simple directions.

Offer food that's too big to put in the mouth, like a full-size sandwich instead of a smaller piece. Trim the crust using a pair of clean kitchen shears, and fringe the edges with each cut about one-half inch apart and about one-half inch deep. Show your toddler how to bite and tear, rather than bite and stuff. When teaching toddlers, a bit of exaggeration always helps! Take a bite yourself and then pull the sandwich away from your body, holding your arm out to the side, far away from your mouth. Say, "Take a bite and take it awayyyyyy!" as you extend your arm and chew. Keep your arm extended until you've swallowed and say, "Let's do it again!" then repeat. Toddlers love this silly game, and it teaches them to slow down, take smaller steps, and tear and chew, rather than stuff and *try to chew.* For kids who don't stuff but just need to practice the bite-and-tear movement, cut the sandwich into triangles, leaving the crust on one side and fringing the other two sides in the same manner. They'll bite off the point and continue to tear off each bite easily if you still say, "Take it awayyyyyy!" Grilled cheese or nut butter and jelly sandwiches work best for this technique, since the cheese and the nut butter stick so well to the bread.

Tricky Transitions:
Breast, Bottles & More

Breast and Bottles

Continue to breastfeed as long as you'd like. There are so many benefits to breastfeeding past the first year, including added nutrition, boosting immunity, and supporting brain development. Balancing breastfeeding and solids by having regularly scheduled meals is crucial to ensure that baby gets a full range of nutrients and continues to develop safe chewing and swallowing skills over the next year.

Drinking from a bottle is mechanically different from breast-feeding, and I recommend weaning from the bottle at the end of the first year. (Please refer to chapter two, page 95.) If your toddler has become attached to the bottle and you're dreading having to bottle-wean, take a deep breath. It's going to be OK! The sooner kids transition from bottles to drinking from cups 100 percent of the time, the easier it will be on everyone.

In chapter two, I discussed how to set up a bottle schedule and gradually shift to eating solids. The most common challenge I hear from parents at baby's first birthday is that their child is "stuck" on nap or bedtime bottles. Kids associate sucking on a bottle and the warmth of the milk with getting sleepy. It's so comforting and relaxing. The key to weaning from the bottle is to include a transition object that baby can associate with comfort and sleep. These "loveys" might be a blanket, stuffed animal, or in the case of one of my little clients, a baseball. He carried that ball everywhere, even to bed. After the age of one year, loveys can be included in the crib.

Offer your toddler a small bottle and the lovey while reading a book or snuggling together just prior to laying them down to sleep. This transition time out of the crib or bed is essential to breaking the tie with having a bottle while lying down. When the bottle is empty, do not refill it. Finish the transition routine and lay your toddler down with the lovey. It's best to quietly remove the bottle from the room. Each day, gradually reduce the amount in the bottle by one or two ounces. Now it's time to eliminate the bottle and replace it with a straw cup. Continue to limit the amount in the cup and, over time, gradually transition to water in the cup. Milk is notorious for creating dental cavities as it pools around the teeth, and water is the ideal drink to have before lying down. Your child will still be comforted, especially if the cup has a short straw for sucking while they get sleepy. Remember, the tip of the straw should reach just the tip of the tongue so that baby can elevate the tongue tip with each swallow. That elevation and pressure from the tongue tip also activates nerves in the alveolar ridge (just above the front teeth) that help kids feel calm. It's one of the reasons kids get hooked on pacifiers and thumb sucking.

Sucking through a straw can be calming

Offering your child thick smoothies or purees with a thin straw provides the oral input that kids crave with sucking. Provide alternatives to sucking on pacifiers, bottles, fingers, or thumbs throughout the day so that when it comes time to wean, it's a much easier process for everyone.

Pacifiers

In chapter two, I shared several strategies for weaning from the pacifier by the end of the first year. If you're still having trouble by 18 months of age, the following three strategies work beautifully for older toddlers:

Sew it up in a lovey. This is an easy method that still keeps the pacifier close for comfort but also keeps it out of your toddler's mouth. Gather all the pacifiers in the house and discard all but one. Choose a favorite lovey (a blanket or stuffed animal) or buy a new one. Using a seam ripper, open a seam and help your child place the paci inside the animal's ear. You can also fold over a corner of a blanket and sew the paci into a pocket there. Sewing machines work best for this purpose, providing a tight stitch to ensure the pacifier stays inside. Now your child can still feel the pacifier, reassured that it's there, and has an extra soft friend to cuddle at night.

Break it, with love. In *Raising a Healthy, Happy Eater*, we described the tried and true "It's broken, can't fix it" method. It's inexpensive and most successful with kids older than 18 months: "Begin by leaving a few broken items around the house, such as a pencil broken in half on the kitchen counter. Pick it up and show it to your toddler, saying, 'Oh, it's broken, can't fix it,' and throw it in the trash. After a week of introducing this concept, take the pacifier that is in the crib and snip off the tip when your child is not there. Discard the tip. Put your child to bed a bit early that day, so that she isn't too tired to encounter the broken pacifier. This is a bittersweet moment to capture on video, because your little one will likely hold up the pacifier and say 'bwoken.' Give her a big hug and take her and the pacifier to the trash can to throw it away."[24] Then, give your toddler another hug, put them in bed again, and parent bravely. You can do it, and so can your toddler.

Enlist the help of the pacifier fairy. The pacifier fairy visits "big kids'" homes and takes their paci to a baby who needs it. However, unlike a tooth for the tooth fairy, the pacifier is not left under the pillow. Help your toddler decorate a large box to leave by the front door of your home. Say goodbye to the last pacifier by placing it in the box, reassuring your toddler that the paci will be going to a tiny baby. Remind your child to check the box in the morning, because the pacifier fairy always leaves a present for big boys and girls who give their pacifier to a new baby who needs it. Don't forget to secretly put that present in the box before you go to bed!

Prior to weaning from the pacifier, remember to offer plenty of other options for chewing and oral input. Kids who rely on pacifiers, or thumb or finger sucking, to calm and focus still need the input to their mouths. Offer teethers that are strong yet flexible, have long pieces to gnaw toward the back of the mouth, and have a wide array of textures. Refer to the appendix, page 215, for ideas on various options. You'll also need to stock up on these if your child is sucking their fingers or thumb.

Thumb and Finger Sucking

The tricky thing about kids who take up thumb or finger sucking is that their tiny digits are always handy and pop so easily into the mouth! Certified orofacial myologists (OFM) are typically SLPs or dental hygienists with intensive advanced training who specialize in eliminating this habit in children starting at age four. Unfortunately, the child's hard palate and dentition, as well as face shape, may already be impacted by consistent digit sucking. Erin Geddes, a certified SLP and OFM, offers the following advice for toddler parents who wish to parent proactively and limit digit sucking early in life[25]:

ADVICE FROM AN EXPERT OROFACIAL MYOLOGIST

Thumb and finger sucking habits can occur for various reasons and are highly associated with airway issues such as allergies, enlarged tonsils and adenoids, medical conditions associated with prematurity, and tethered oral tissues, also known as tongue-, lip-, and cheek-ties. It is important to begin the process of ruling out why the sucking habit has occurred and find a few creative ways to decrease the intensity, frequency, and duration of the sucking habit, which can have effects on the teeth, the formation of the roof of the mouth into a normal U shape, and the development of a mature swallow pattern during early childhood.

The goal is to begin replacing the sucking habit with age-appropriate activities that encourage the tongue, cheeks, lips, and jaw to work in various positions to promote a balanced orofacial development. Sucking places the tongue in a low, forward position so that it is not resting at the proper spot in the mouth. The proper spot in the mouth is at the incisive papilla, the spot right behind the upper, central incisors. (That's the spot we use to make the /d/ sound.) There is a nerve bundle on that spot known as the trigeminal nerve and it's chock-full of receptors. These receptors cause the release of the neurotransmitters responsible for self-soothing, concentration, and mood control, and help promote sleep. The release of these neuro-transmitters occurs when your child sucks on their thumb or fingers. When your child sucks, they are obtaining positive feedback from the sucking, and that feedback is what makes it so addicting and hard to stop.

To assist in minimizing your child's sucking habit, try the following:

- Determine the frequency: How often and at what times of the day and night are they sucking?

- Determine the duration: How long they are sucking?

- Determine the intensity: How hard they are sucking on their digits?

- Take note of what is happening right before they begin to suck. Are they also using a blanket, a favorite stuffed animal, tags from clothing, toys, or blankets when they are sucking?

- Once you've determined the above, then begin to change up the child's routine:

- If they are sucking during car rides, have them play a game to keep them awake.

- Do not let them watch a movie or have an iPad if that is a time they suck on their thumbs or fingers. Instead sing silly songs together or play a car game such as I Spy.

- Changing the child's routine includes their sleep routine. Prior to going to sleep, provide extra cuddle time, listen to soothing music, and increase reading time. This is also when you would eliminate the stuffed animal or blanket that is associated with the sucking habit. Please note that this is different from eliminating the pacifier, as described earlier in this chapter. Because the pacifier can be removed from the scene (and a thumb cannot) the transition object provides comfort instead of the pacifier. When the object is associated with sucking on thumbs or fingers, it's best to fade out the presence of the object.

Oral input can be included throughout the day to help your toddler get the input they crave without relying on thumb or digit sucking. Add tongue brushing to your child's toothbrushing routine. Brush the sides of the tongue from back to front. Brush the middle of the tongue from back to front. Brush the tongue tip. Then go up to the roof of the mouth right behind the top teeth and brush up there with a nice U shape to give some input where the thumb was pressing in the past. It's always fun to sing a song while brushing so your child knows the start and end time. When the song is over, always stop brushing to build trust, especially if your child doesn't tolerate toothbrushing well. Remember to provide regular access to teethers or safe chewy toys for oral exploration as an alternative to the oral input that they got from digit sucking.

Teach toddlers to spit out that toothpaste!

Kids under the age of three should have the tiniest bit of toothpaste on the toothbrush, no bigger than a grain of rice. By age three, pediatric dentists allow a pea-size dab on the brush. Regardless of the amount, toddlers will build up saliva as you're helping them brush, and they will need to spit. While your child is standing on a step stool at the bathroom sink, follow the Three Ts method (Toothpaste, Target, Two!) to teach kids ages two and older how to spit into the sink:

Toothpaste: Just a little bit!

Target: A sticker or any target works as long as it stays in place in the sink. Ideally, draw the number two on the target, with the number facing your child so they can see it.

Two: When your little one is ready to spit, encourage them to enthusiastically say, "TWO," with a little force on their tongue. Because they are looking at the target, seeing the visual cue "2," and are tilting their head down, they can't help but spit. With a little practice, they will become more proficient at it, but expect a little mess at first!

There have been so many transitions to navigate in these quick six months! Your child is now on a consistent meal- and snack-time feeding schedule and using cups and utensils! Biting, chewing, and manipulating food from table to mouth is purposeful, with little to no reliance on oral reflexes. You're offering a variety of safe foods to continue to build oral-motor skills and for balanced nutrition. Bottles and pacifiers are now a thing of the past. But what's most obvious is that your child has a personality and temperament all their own, unique in every way! That's something to celebrate and embrace, especially as your child gains momentum toward the Terrific Twos.

Chapter Four

Rounding the Bend

· 18 TO 24 MONTHS ·

As toddlers are rounding the bend and approaching the terrific twos, you will observe significant changes in both feeding and language development. It will require a keen eye and a bit of detective work to decipher exactly what your child is trying to tell you. Your toddler is using 25 words or more to express wants and needs, waving bye-bye, and playing finger games like itsy-bitsy spider (even if they can't say the entire rhyme). Animal sounds are exceedingly popular, and when your toddler says, "Mooooo!" it may indicate that they spotted a cow in the nearby field rather than the sound the cow makes. At this stage, if your 18-month-old is not uttering at least ten words while doing any of the following, be sure to consult with your pediatrician. All attempts at communication count! Examples include:

- Word approximations (*Mah* for *Mom*)
- Exclamatory words (*Yayyyyyy!*)
- Sign language with no vocalizations

- Animal sounds or signs for animals
- Gestures (waving bye)

Toddlers understand more than they can verbalize, and they can follow one-step directions, such as "Give me the spoon, please." They may be saying some words ("more") rather than signing. By age two, you will witness a spurt in language development as your toddler's vocabulary reaches at least 50 single words and they begin putting two words together. Many children achieve this milestone before their second birthday.

Language Development during Mealtimes

You can help drive expressive language development specifically during meals or with your child in the kitchen. Cooking with toddlers can be so fun (and, yes, messy!), and it's an interactive way to boost along your toddler's communication skills. Speech pathologist Grace Bernales offers the following tips for both meals and cooking times with toddlers[1]:

> "Sabotaging" is a technique used by SLPs that simply means setting your child up for success with open-ended scenarios for speech and language. For example, rather than giving your toddler a full glass of milk, give them only a small amount. That way, your toddler can request more by producing a single word and/or sign language like "more" or "milk." If your toddler is already producing two- to three-word phrases, they can request by producing, "I want more" or "more milk." This isn't the time to insist on your child talking, but it is the time to provide opportunities for conversations.[2]
>
> In addition, "sabotaging" during the cooking process can increase your toddler's opportunity to request. For instance, you can pretend you gave them the wrong cookware or place the desired object (e.g., ingredient, plastic bowl, spatula) out of reach, so that your toddler can produce the word or sign "help." It's important to remember not to always anticipate your child's needs, so that they are more likely to ask for assistance, whether you're cooking or eating.[3]

"Say _____" is the last thing you want to say!

One of the very first things SLPs learn in their training is to stop using the phrase "Say (doggie, cat, mommy, milk, and so on)." Communication is not based on drill or route motor practice. Like responsive feeding, conversations are reciprocal, with a back-and-forth flow that allows for each person to initiate a turn. When parents prompt kids to say a word by using the phrase "Say _____" the reciprocity is lost, the meaning is not purposeful for communication, and the child relies on the parent to initiate each language performance.

Labeling nouns: Mealtimes are perfect for teaching commonly used nouns (e.g., for food, drink, utensils), labeling each while eating. Make sure to emphasize these nouns multiple times (e.g., "You're eating an apple, that's an apple, mmm apple!"), as this is important for exposure to new vocabulary. Many different verbs are also utilized when eating, which you can narrate as the action is happening. If you're pouring water, you can say, "pour, pour, pour!" or "pouring water." While your toddler is chewing their food, rather than just watching them, you can say "chew, chew, chew" or say a short phrase like "You're chewing chicken."[4]

As you're cooking the ingredients, you can narrate your actions by labeling the verbs, nouns, prepositions, and/or adjectives (e.g., "mix, mix, mix," "pour oil," "ooh, hot," "in pan"). Exclamatory sounds or words (e.g., "oooooh," "wow," "yummm," "mmmmm," "ahhhhh," "whoa!") are easier for toddlers to imitate. Have them imitate action (e.g., blow/fan the food when it's hot, stir the ingredients).

Boosting receptive language, such as following simple one-step directions, fits nicely into mealtime routines. When your toddler is all done eating, you can model the words and/or sign "all done" and then have them follow directions like "give me the cup" or "wipe your mouth," and so on.

If you have an older toddler, you can ask more complex questions, like "Where is the green vegetable?" or follow directions with attributes (e.g., "Get the *big, orange* fruit").

Mealtimes are not a quiz show

Asking questions is a part of our normal conversations, but bombarding kids with too many questions can backfire by shutting down a child's attempts at communication and adding unintended pressure at mealtimes. Limit questions to no more than 20 percent of the interactions and use them as a tool to help the conversation continue.

Symbolic Play

Pioneering child psychologist Jean Piaget once said, "Play is the answer to how anything new comes about," and this is true for your child's discovery of new words and new foods. It's a vital component of cognitive development. By now, your two-year-old has begun to engage in symbolic play, and you'll notice it throughout the day. When in the kitchen, the wooden spoon might suddenly transform into a telephone as your toddler puts it up to his ear and pretends to call Grandma to tell her what you're baking together. At mealtimes, penne pasta becomes a trumpet as they "toot-toot" through the tube of pasta throughout dinner! Unless it's becoming too much of a distraction and you feel the need to redirect, try to embrace these playful moments. Your toddler is practicing problem solving, expressing their feelings via this pretend play, and learning about symbols. Early symbolic play is the foundation for understanding numbers and letters and, ultimately, learning to read. Use your own imagination to model all the possibilities: Green beans might transform into two walrus tusks emerging from under your top lip, or a bread stick might become a fairy wand. When we respond to our children's playful communication, that connection is priceless and always memorable.

Just like the surge in language skills, feeding development blossoms during the latter part of the second year. Every aspect of fine-motor development has matured, and kids are ready for larger utensils, can spear food with a fork with ease, and can learn the basics of cutting with a child-safe knife. Even their chewing pattern changes as they learn to move their jaw in more of a circular motion, called a rotary chew. Kids can hold pieces of toast or larger crackers and intentionally bite off pieces with significant control, grading the amount of pressure they apply to two different textures, like a quesadilla versus a crunchy cookie. By age two, kids have mastered open-cup drinking and may only spill when they accidentally knock over a cup or are distracted. From the period of 18 to 24 months, there are specific strategies to ensure that kids reach these feeding milestones, building skill and ability in the process.

Building More Skill & Ability for Self-Feeding

Mastering Open-Cup Drinking

In chapter two, I shared tips for offering tiny cups of purees or liquids to help baby learn to sip from an open cup. Learning to hold a cup steady without spilling isn't typically mastered until toddlers are closer to 24 months old, but once your toddler can follow simple one- to two-step directions, you can help them master open-cup drinking using my Magic 1, 2, 3, 4 Method[5]:

> The key to teaching a child to drink from an open cup is to break it into simple steps and master one skill at a time. Choose a small cup (see appendix, page 215, for suggestions) or—for an inexpensive alternative—a small, glass baby food jar or two- to four-ounce canning jar. The glass on these jars is so thick that they truly don't break that easily. For added grip, tightly wrap a few wide rubber bands around the glass. The small jars are the ideal size for little hands, and the mouth of the jar is the perfect

circumference to fit in the corners of a toddler's mouth. Too often, parents use their own adult-size glass to offer sips to a child, but think about it—that's like you and me drinking from a bucket. Fill the jar with water to where the lid of the jar screws on. Thanks to the weight of it when filled almost to the brim, kids can feel the cup in their hands, and that weight helps send signals to the brain via the sense of proprioception. Add a splash of color with a dark-colored juice so your child can easily see the surface of the water.

Now, you're ready to teach four simple steps to drinking from an open cup:

- Magic Step #1: Using hand-over-hand guidance or by modeling with your own cup, help your child lift the cup straight up from the table and set it back down. Practice several times, repeating the mantra, "Lift up, set down, stay dry."

- Magic Step #2: Add a new step to the end of this sequence. Bring the cup to the child's lips and have them sip, but not tilt. Your toddler will be able to do this because she can see the surface of the water and it's filled high enough that there is no need to tip. Your child may have practiced tipping before (and pouring water down the front of their shirt). The mantra and sequence are now "Lift up, cup to lips, sip, set down, stay dry." Practice as many times as needed, replenishing the water to ensure there is no need to tilt the cup.

- Magic Step #3: Now you're ready to teach the tilt-up, and, more important, if you want to avoid a waterfall, it's time to teach the tilt-down. Kids who spent months drinking from a sippy cup have trouble with this stage, because they are used to sipping and then pulling the cup away without immediately tipping it back down. But, because you rarely ever used a sippy cup, your toddlers won't have that issue! To teach the tilt-down, you should encourage your child to bring the cup to their chest. (I refer to this area as the

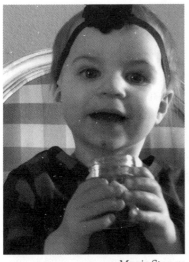

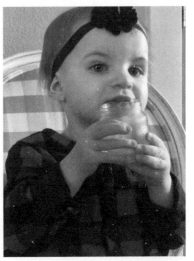

Magic Step #1

Magic Step #2

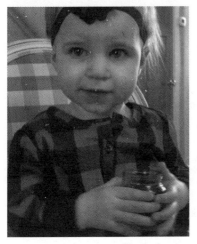

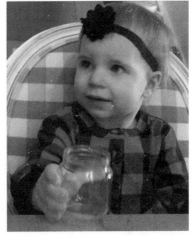

Magic Step #3

Magic Step #4

"tummy" since young toddlers seem to think that "tummy" means anything between shoulders and hips, but it's fine to say "chest" if that works with your older child.) Say, "Put your cup on your tummy," pointing to your entire chest and belly area. Now the mantra and sequence are as follows: "Lift up, cup to lips, sip, cup on your tummy." Repeat several times, but don't refill the glass. As the surface of the liquid lowers with each sip, your child will naturally tilt the glass slightly to sip. The key is the step "Put the cup on your tummy," which automatically causes the child to tilt the cup down.

- Magic Step #4: Once your toddler has learned to put the edge of the cup on their tummy, they can either rest it there until drinking again or follow through by placing it back on the table. That fourth and final step causes the cup to rest or be raised up again to repeat the sequence. Now your toddler is drinking from a cup—and with minimal spills!

When we break down motor tasks into small steps and then chain them into a sequence, kids learn to pay attention to each individual step. They watch the cup more closely; they feel the weight of the cup better; and they get the best possible feedback from the muscles, joints, and brain to signal "Well done! You did it!"

Transitioning to Bigger Utensils

Graduating to larger utensils might feel a little scary when kids have been waving around plastic or silicone spoons for months! The decision to move to stainless steel or any utensil with firm, pointy tines on the fork is best made after asking three questions:

1. Is my child's mouth large enough for this bigger spoon and fork?
2. Does my child have the attention and motor skills to use more advanced utensils?
3. Is it necessary and helpful?

Bigger utensils are meant for bigger bodies, hands, and mouths. A larger spoon or fork will often deliver a larger amount of food with each bite. The widths of the spoon and the fork need to fit comfortably in a child's mouth without their having to struggle to open their mouth enough to take in the utensil and the food all at once. Shop for a stainless set that has a built-up plastic handle that is slightly thicker than an adult utensil. The part of the spoon or fork that enters the mouth is often constructed of stainless steel. The "mouth pieces" should be slightly larger than the toddler utensils you've been offering in the past, but not as large as a typical adult's utensils.

The tines of the fork should have a slightly rounded point at the end to pierce foods without hurting gums or lips that may accidentally encounter a tine as toddlers are learning. This is why motor skills need to be age-appropriate at the 18- to 24-month level. By now, your toddler can[6]:

- feed themselves with smaller plastic or silicone utensils
- turn pages in a book one at a time
- place pegs in a pegboard
- build towers of four or more blocks
- scribble and try to draw lines up, down, and across a page, as well as circles

Attention is still fleeting at this age. Every toddler should eat sitting down and buckled into their feeding chair. A quick tumble or a sudden urge to stand with a stainless utensil in hand can result in serious injury.

The knife in your utensil set should have a rounded point and be blunt enough not to cut skin. The handle should be thick, ideally with a guard for a little fist to brace against and to prevent toddlers from holding the metal part of the knife by mistake. At this stage, the knife is less likely to be used at the mealtime table and more likely to be for helping in the kitchen. However, with softer foods like noodles, it's fine to include a child-safe knife to spark interest, especially in a new food at mealtimes.

Occupational therapist (OT) Mia McCloy explains the necessary fine motor skills for cutting, and how they emerge over time: "Kids need to be able to have finger isolation of the index finger and then good stabilization of the rest of the fingers to stabilize the knife in their palm while they cut [at mealtimes]."[7] Once those skills are emerging, they can start practicing cutting bite sizes of soft foods on their plate. Parents will see more consistency as their fine-motor skills get stronger. With practice, knife skills continue to develop as your child enters kindergarten, with mastery achieved in elementary school.

Learning to Use a Knife

Older toddlers can learn to cut soft foods while you prep meals in the kitchen. Be sure they are in a safety learning tower or bring their high chair into the kitchen for them to sit and practice. Their "cutting hand" grasps the handle of the knife in their fist, and the point of the knife is kept down on the cutting board. Use your hand to show them how to rock the knife. Thin strips of cucumber or jicama are perfect for practice, and if they pop a piece in their mouth, that's a bonus! Teach them how to hold the cucumber spear with their fingertips tucked under their knuckles, like a cat paw. That kitty-paw grasp protects tiny fingers from an accidental squish with the knife. It won't cut them, but the squish of metal would hurt!

Mealtime Transitions: The Beginning and End of the Meal

Toddlers sometimes have difficulty with transitions, moving from one activity to another. Providing a gentle heads-up by saying, "In a few minutes, we're going to clean up the toys and have a yummy lunch" or a similar script to share that a new activity will be starting soon is always helpful. Marking the beginning of any special activity helps toddlers get into the groove of what's about to happen next. At mealtimes, once all of the food is ready to be served, mark the beginning of the meal with a simple prayer, a short song, or a routine in which your toddler can be an active participant. By age two, kids can even help light a small candle with you as you hold the match and they hold your wrist as you place the votive container in the center of the table. These family traditions that open the meal signify that this is a special time!

Likewise, marking the end of a meal helps kids say, "I'm all done" and closes the door on eating time. There will be no more food available for a few hours, following the meal- and snack-time schedule guidelines outlined on page 69. Toddlers can sing a cleanup song or blow out the candle. Create your own family tradition with a silly handshake or a family fist bump to signal "That was a fun meal!" Starting when your toddler is about 18 months of age, teach them to take their plate to the kitchen, even if they can't quite reach high enough to place it on the counter. You can do that part for them or show them where to set it on a stool or shelf beneath the countertop for you to clear later. In Montessori education, kids as young as two scrape their plates and help wash them! The end-of-meal routine of taking our own plates to the kitchen helps the transition from eating time to growing time go smoothly. Toddlers thrive on predictability and routine.

It's astounding what our toddlers can do! I asked Nancy Creskoff Maune, a pediatric OT at Children's Hospital Colorado, to share the progression of development that leads to something as surprising as a young toddler helping to clear the table[8]:

- 9 to 12 months old: Most babies start walking at this age, and most learn to walk well in the months after their first birthday.

- 13 to 14 months old: After walking for a few months, toddlers develop a more mature gait, holding their hands at their sides (rather than up or out in front for balance) and moving with their feet closer together. Toddlers learn to turn, start, and stop without losing their balance. Your child will begin to feel more confident about walking and will take on new challenges— such as stooping to pick up objects, moving while pulling a toy behind, and walking on uneven surfaces.

- 15 to 18 months old: At this age, children can imitate simple household tasks and chores, and they will begin to practice walking while holding something in their arms. Carrying a large toy or item with two hands is a milestone in development that emerges between 17 and 18.5 months of age, according to the *Hawaii Early Learning Profile* developmental assessment tool.

You may want to practice outside of mealtimes by having your child carry a medium-size ball or large stuffed toy with two hands, and then show them how to carry a tray or a hardback book with one hand on each side so that it remains (fairly) flat. Once your toddler has mastered walking while carrying, have them clear the dishes and cups that are empty of food and liquid and that are not breakable, for best success and safety. You can scrape what's left of their meal onto your plate before handing them the dirty plate to carry to the kitchen.

- 24 months old: Children typically begin to be able to stand on tiptoes for a few seconds. With time and practice, your child will become more coordinated and may be able to reach up to the sink or place items on the countertop.

Toddlers love to help, and it's daily activities like these—with transitions from one activity to the next—that build gross- and fine-motor skills while working on balance and body awareness. One of the best things that Nancy taught me when I was a new clinician over twenty years ago was "Let them do it themselves." When kids get to experience all their skills and abilities without our stepping in to do it for them, they gain confidence and trust in the world. Adults are there to support and guide our children to participate in all aspects of the day, even clearing the table, as long as they are capable.

How long does it take for kids to eat?

On average, toddlers can learn to sit at a table for fifteen to twenty minutes max. If they get squirmy before then and need to get down, it's understandable! They probably aren't that hungry, and responsive feeding means that we honor a child's hunger and satiety cues. Rather than watching the clock, watch your child, and you'll know when it's time for them to get down. On the rare occasion when you feel that mealtimes are lasting too long, give a verbal reminder like "Let's finish our lunch, it's time for playground time!" and help your child take their plate to the counter. There is always more food coming, and sticking to a reasonable schedule will help a child tune in to internal cues to eat or not.

Napkins: Yay or Nay?

Kids as young as 18 months can have a small napkin beside them at the table, if it doesn't become a distraction. Some children prefer a slightly damp, gentle "baby" washcloth for added texture and ease of cleaning. They can use it on their own periodically, following your lead as you show them how you use a napkin on your own face or hands. But when it comes time to clean up their messy hands and face, if they are opposed, try not to wipe them down while they're still seated at the table. Lift them out of the chair (use the extended arm hold to keep yourself clean) and let them wash at the sink instead. Many toddlers are tactically averse to napkins or washcloths, especially on their face. They still need to get cleaned up, but move the unpleasantness away from the table so they don't associate it with eating. Try different textures and softnesses to see which they prefer and take advantage of running water, which most kids adore. Then it's a quick pat dry and they're off to play!

Try This for Sensitive Faces!

Many children dislike having their face washed because of the way we rub across their lips and cheeks. Instead of randomly stroking in any direction, do one side and then the other. Their nose is "midline," and you never want to cross there. Instead, using a firm, steady pressure, wipe from the center of their lips, again at midline, and stroke outward toward their ear. Stop and return to that same spot, stroking in the same direction until the face is clean. Repeat on the other side. Sing a song or make some silly sound effects with each wipe. Close your eyes and have someone wipe your face in random directions. It's so dysregulating to the nervous system! When kids have predictability in their cleanup routine, they can tolerate the sensation over time.

Teach toddlers that they can use a napkin to politely and safely spit out anything that's uncomfortable in their mouth. Adults experience this from time to time. We bite into a stringy piece of meat or a peculiar soft spot in an apple, and we calmly reach for the napkin in our lap to expel the offending food. If kids don't feel comfortable chewing or swallowing, they always have permission to remove food politely from their mouths.

Provide water with a thin straw to help kids wash down small pieces of chewed food or to rinse their mouth after placing the distasteful piece in the napkin. A thin straw delivers less water to the tongue and provides just enough moisture to propel the food back, rather than have it float behind the lips. As long as it's not spoiled, learning to swallow less tasteful food and rinsing with water is a skill I teach early in life.

Model how to use a napkin at the table, intentionally and quietly removing a chewed piece of food when your child is watching. Occasionally reach for a sip of water to help wash down chewed food, too. You really are the best teacher!

Teaching the Intentional Swallow

By 18 months of age, your toddler has the cognitive ability to learn exactly what "swallow" means and to do it on command. But parents need to teach the concept in a simple, fun, and visual way. The following method teaches kids what it means when "food goes in your tummy."

You will need:

- A tube sock and a marker or felt to make eyes, lips, and a nose. Add yarn for hair and some ears if you're feeling very crafty!
- A long-sleeve shirt, with sleeves that fit tightly on your forearm.
- Large poker chips or child-safe pretend food shaped like a thin cookie.

Directions:

1. Make a sock puppet, cutting a small slit where the puppet fits into the palm of your hand. That will represent the back of the puppet's throat.

2. Put the puppet on your hand, extending the longer part of the sock down your forearm.

3. Pull the sleeve of your shirt *over* the sock on your arm.

4. Bend your arm at the elbow and let your toddler feed the puppet "cookies" (the large poker chips or pretend food noted above). As the puppet chews and swallows, the cookie can be seen going down your sleeve and will stop at the bend of your elbow. Each time a cookie is swallowed, the bulge near your elbow will get bigger. That's the puppet's tummy!

5. Say "chew chew" with each chewing motion, then "swallow" as the cookie goes down the throat/sleeve. Let your toddler push the puppet's belly as you say, "Oh, he's getting full! Lots of cookies down in his belly! He swallowed the cookie! It's in his belly!" This type of repetition is what helps build language and the concept of "swallow."

6. Later, repeat the same verbal cues while eating. Use "chew" and "swallow" and "down to my tummy," allowing your toddler to place their hands on the front of your throat to feel the swallow. Toddlers can also gently feel their own swallow with sips of water or food over time.

> ### What is a swallow?
>
> Teaching kids the concept and mechanics of swallowing is helpful as they learn to taste new foods, learn how to spit out toothpaste (and not swallow it), and when explaining why small toys or other nonfood objects like coins don't go in our mouth. Swallow is an abstract concept in general, but using a playful method to help them visualize what's happening when food "goes to the tummy" helps kids apply it to many different scenarios.

Travel Cups

Cups for day care, trips to the park, and other outings need special features to keep drinks warm or cool, and they need to be relatively spill-proof. Whether your preference is stainless steel or a plastic insulated container, the lid should be easy to open and shut so kids can do it on their own. A pop-up straw is easiest, and the lid should cover it completely when it closes to keep the drinking area clean. Some cups may have valves embedded in the tip of the straw or farther down the length of the straw to prevent spilling. However, valves can make straws tricky for toddlers, causing them to have to brace and bite on the straw to extract the liquid. That bracing is discouraged by speech pathologists, since it's not part of typical drinking development and may create overuse and distortions of facial musculature. I suggest avoiding hard plastic or wide rectangular pop-up straws, as these also encourage bracing with the teeth. If your child can drink easily without bracing, you've found a good travel cup! Consider how tall the travel cup is, too. For example, when it is placed on a restaurant table with your child seated, the straw should barely reach the tip of the nose or below. Toddlers will need to hold the cup and tilt it to drink, and when the straw reaches above the tip of the nose, that's almost impossible.

Avoid stainless steel bottles that have a narrow neck and a screw-off cap for drinking (like from an open cup). There have been incidences of children inadvertently putting their tongue inside the neck of the bottle while drinking, creating suction, and getting their tongue stuck inside. Some of these do have narrow, flip-up straws, but never allow your child to drink directly from the neck of the bottle. Some of my favorite travel cups are listed in the appendix.

Feeding & Communication Myths

Using a divided plate creates picky eaters.
Use a variety of plates, some divided, some not. Both have advantages. Divided plates keep foods that roll or sauces that run contained. The barriers make it easier for kids to brace little fingers as they try to pick up a pea or a yummy rice ball. Ice cube trays and muffin tins are another form of divided plates, both fantastic for increasing variety in each section and offering a smorgasbord as a meal. However, when kids become dependent on divided plates, they fuss over foods touching and can become rigid about what foods go in each section. Rotate through all the options—that's the key!

Once my toddler has learned to chew, I don't need to cut foods anymore.
Cut foods for safe swallowing until age four. I cannot emphasize this enough. Toddlers are still perfecting the motor movements for chewing, and they have limited attention spans. Combining immature motor skills and fleeting attention spans with a very narrow airway easily leads to choking episodes if we aren't careful. By age

four, kids have mastered the motor skills, improved their attention, and developed a slightly larger airway. Like adults, there is still a possibility for choking, but the risk is reduced.

Drooling in toddlers is common.

Drooling in toddlers happens periodically when they are teething or sick. However, constant drooling is *not* common in typically developing kids and requires an evaluation by an SLP or OT who specializes in oral motor development in children. Toddlers who drool consistently day after day may need intervention due to low muscle tone, open mouth and forward tongue posture, and more.

All my kids used sippy cups and pacifiers, and they turned out fine.

Sucking has an impact on facial formation, and this includes breastfeeding. However, the breast is designed to support the development of the palate and the adjoining structures of the face as a child grows. Finger sucking, pacifiers, and spouted sippy cups alter that formation, but the degree of alteration is always dependent on how hard the child sucks, how frequently they suck, and how long they maintain the suck. This intensity, frequency, and duration, along with multifactorial habits like breathing through the mouth (and not the nose), always influence facial formation to some degree. My own children had pacifiers for too long, and I didn't see a problem with it because at the time I wasn't trained to see how it might influence their facial features. One child ended up with braces, and the other did not. Today, I know better and hope to educate parents around the world on the importance of healthy mouth development.

My toddler isn't talking much, but lots of kids are late talkers.

There is some indication that some children catch up with language development with their peers by age five. But is it worth the risk to wait it out? ASHA states that late talkers "may be at risk for developing language and/or literacy difficulties as they age." Like delays in feeding development, any gap in speech and language development needs to be brought to the attention of your pediatrician. Discuss what you're observing with your child's doctor to determine the best course of action for your family.[9]

My toddler is waking up hungry at night.

Unless there is a metabolic or medical reason for waking with hunger pangs, it's not common for hunger to be the culprit when kids have trouble staying asleep. If a child has a meal or a snack within an hour of the bedtime routine, they have enough in their belly to feel comfortably full all night. When kids wake in the middle of the night and ask for food, it's best to let your pediatrician know of this habit, just to rule out possible medical causes. Keep a spill-proof cup of water by your toddler's bed that's easy to reach in case of thirst.

My toddler needs their thumb/bottle/pacifier for comfort.

Feeling like a bad parent for taking away what comforts your child most, like the pacifier? Reframe your thinking: Children begin to learn to self-soothe without pacifiers as early as 6 months, and your little one is more than capable of that, too. Weaning from a dependence on sucking for comfort isn't always easy, but the sooner you do, the better everyone will be for it. After the first year, kids get the oral input they need from eating solid foods and sucking from straws. During the transition phase, they may need teethers or chewies to provide some oral input. Repeated sucking on a pacifier, bottle, or thumb can change the formation of your child's beautiful face. Parent bravely. You can do it.

Chapter Five

Coasting through Challenges

• 24 TO 36 MONTHS •

You are about to enter a parent's most dreaded stage of raising a toddler: The Terrible Twos. There's no reason to panic! This chapter is devoted to helping you coast through the most common challenges at this age, starting with understanding why toddlers love one word the most, and that word is no.

Responding to Your Toddler's No

One of the first words that your toddler learned prior to turning two is no, and now they'll test it out with a vengeance! A two-year-old's cognitive development is centered around discovering their independence. You will observe them having strong opinions, making decisive choices that may make no sense to an adult, and their behavior can feel rigid at times. Meanwhile, language development is also taking flight, with kids speaking in full sentences by age three. The toddler's burst in cognition, the striving for independence, and the ever-expanding receptive and expressive language skills are why this stage in life can be so challenging for adults. When kids are more equipped to test their environment, parents need to stay one step ahead.

Although toddlers understand more concepts, such as definers of time ("after dinner"), they may not always cooperate and be able to wait. They also don't understand nuances such as "I'm going to eat your mac-n-cheese before you do" and may interpret good-natured teasing as the rock-solid truth, leading to outbursts and tantrums out of frustration.

During this period of rapid brain growth, toddlers begin to grasp the concept that they are uniquely different beings than their parents. They quickly learn that they have considerable control over your actions and behaviors. Still, they crave boundaries to feel safe, and that's why the word no may be one of their favorites. It's a very delicate time in a child's emotional development.

Armed with the knowledge of all that your toddler is going through, it's easier to parent compassionately when kids take a strong stand and refuse to eat or even come to the table. Offering choices is the best way to deflect their stance and shape more positive behaviors. Toddlers like to choose between two options, in which case, answering no just doesn't make sense to them. However, be aware that most toddlers will pick the second choice, because it's the last option they heard and processed before answering you. That can work to your advantage if you're really hoping they pick carrots in the example that follows. But, if your toddler wanted broccoli, they'll definitely object when you hand them the carrot! Responding to kids' sometimes fickle attempts at communication requires parenting patiently, so try again—and this time, reverse the two choices to ensure that you're responding to their true preference:

"We have broccoli or carrots today. Which one would you like on your plate?"

"It's time for lunch! Red plate or blue plate, which do you want?"

Responding to Big Emotions with the ABCs

Two-year-olds have big feelings and big emotions, sometimes over the littlest things! Tantrums are bound to happen, but how you respond can make all the difference in helping toddlers feel secure. Emotional outbursts are most often due to a child's frustration over their limited ability to express their wants and needs. Truthfully, they sometimes don't even know themselves what they want and need. They just know *this* (whatever "this" is—the wrong size chicken nugget, the wrong color plate, or the wrong princess on the cup) is *not* OK, and they're demanding that you fix it . . . *now*.

Take a breath and remember my ABCs when responding:

A: Acknowledge the feelings. When kids refuse what you've offered, acknowledge their feelings so they feel heard and supported in their communication attempt.

- "You're feeling mad about these chicken nuggets. You wanted the dinosaur-shape nuggets."

B: Brave boundaries! Maintain your boundaries and parent bravely.

- "Today, we have the round nuggets."

C: Choices help kids feel in control of their emotions. Offer a choice of a condiment or side dish to help them feel some control.

- "We need a dip, too. Would you like ketchup or honey?"

Here are a few more examples:

A: "You're frustrated that we don't have crackers for breakfast. It's OK to feel that way."

B: "We'll have crackers today when we visit the zoo."

C: "Which lunchbox should we put the crackers in, the one with the picture of the truck or the one with the elephant?"

A: "You're sad that mealtime ended, and you want to get back in your chair."

B: "Now it's playing time. We'll have more food after we play outside."

C: "Do you want to play in the backyard or go to the park?"

Parenting consistently means sticking to strategies, even if you encounter loud complaints from your toddler no matter what you do. Just state the ABCs once and move on. Stay calm, keep your response concise (A, B, C, and done!), and maintain that consistent behavior with every new tantrum. It won't take long to see the change in your toddler. The magnitude and duration of each emotional outburst will diminish each day until they are less frequent and less intense.

Responsive Play

Just like responsive feeding, think of any type of social play as responsive play. Playing with others helps children learn to notice social cues, listen, and consider another person's perspective. These are all key elements of developing empathy. According to Harvard University's Graduate School of Education: "Especially in social and guided play, children learn self-regulation as they follow norms and pay attention while experiencing feelings such as anticipation or frustration."[1]

Responding to Cries for Food

It happens in every household. Twenty minutes before dinner will be ready, the kids start saying, "But I'm so hungry!" Today, everything seems to happen so quickly for kids. Their favorite television show pops up on the screen just by talking into the remote. They can call Grandma just by touching her picture on a screen. (When I was a kid, I couldn't call my grandmother because I wasn't old enough to memorize a phone number and it cost extra to call "long distance." I had to wait till the weekends, when my parents would help me and it was cheaper.) I know three-year-olds who have bought toys on Amazon.com just by clicking the Buy Now with 1-Click button on a touch screen before their parents had a chance to stop them. So, life is cool for kids, but "waiting" has become a lost art.

In earlier chapters, we've discussed the importance of sticking to a consistent meal and snack time schedule. But when I had two kids under the age of three, some days I needed less fussing about "When's dinner?!!!!" and more peace and quiet so I could get dinner on the table.

What do you do when you don't want to spoil their appetite, yet you don't want to listen to the fussing while you're rushing to prepare a meal? Try a nibble tray.

The Nibble Tray

When hungry is turning into "hangry," parent proactively. Have an ice cube tray in your fridge, preloaded with tiny pieces of fruit or protein. You can add a few bites of whatever you're trying to get on the dinner table, too, like a piece of steamed broccoli. You don't have to put food in every space in your ice cube tray, but tossing a few pieces of cereal or a small cracker in each space around the other selections is fine, too. Each square in the tray shouldn't have more than a small piece or two of a fruit, vegetable, carb, or protein. It's for nibbling, and is not a replacement for dinner. Think of it as a healthy appetizer. No refills, please. Parent consistently and stick to that rule, no matter what. The best thing about a nibble tray is that it's easy to assemble in less than a minute, or you can have one already in the fridge for moments of "starvation." Didn't need it? Just cover and save it in case you need it tomorrow.

Parent Mindfully

A consistent meal- and snack-time schedule may occasionally include an appetizer or nibble tray *if children ask for it*. But nibble trays don't appear every time a child says they're hungry throughout the day. As toddlers get older, requests to eat before scheduled eating times may often just be a response to thirst or boredom or a need for your attention. Even with a few years of responsive feeding practice, kids will still be kids! Like adults, they don't always read their body's needs perfectly, and often they can wait. A tall glass of cool water and a hug may be all they need.

The Natural Fear of New Foods

Why are so many toddlers so picky? We've discussed how growth slows down after age one and even more after age two. Kids are moving more and exploring the power of no! Some research refers to the period between 18 months and three years when kids have a natural fear of new foods as neophobia. However, the term neophobia is also used to refer to extreme picky eating behaviors that require feeding therapy. It's a confusing term, because in some literature it refers to a natural phase and in other studies, a need for intervention. Some factors, such as pressure to eat, temperament, parental practices or feeding styles, and social influences, sensory preferences, and food culture will have similar effects on both magnitude and duration of fussy eating.

How, then, can parents practice responsive feeding strategies and rest assured that this natural phase of more hesitant eating is simply the core of toddler eating behavior? In chapter seven, I'll share red flags to watch out for if you suspect your child may need extra support from a feeding specialist. Early intervention is key any time a child appears to be stalling in feeding development or appears stressed or fearful about eating. Excessive fussiness has been associated with the diagnosis of failure to thrive when a child's growth stalls significantly as compared to peers who are the same age and sex.

> TIP: Ban the term "picky eater" from your house. Although it's a term I use in all of my articles and books, it's a label I avoid using in front of a child. Kids will always live up to the labels we assign to them. All children are learning eaters (and most adults are, too!) or food explorers!

Family-Style Strategies

Gathering around the table and helping ourselves to bowls of vegetables, a basket of rolls, and a platter of freshly carved turkey is referred to as family-style serving. We often pass the bowls and platters from person to person, and everyone takes whatever they would like. It's a lovely way to share a meal! However, it does require a bit more work, adds a few more dirty dishes that need cleaning, and it isn't easy or safe for children under the age of three to handle heavy or hot containers of food.

Instead, try my "master server" and "big scoop, small sample" strategy. Kids as young as two can do this with your help, and by age three they will truly be a master server! The serving bowls and platters are placed in front of the master server. Then, each family member passes their plate up to where the master server is seated and requests a big scoop or a small sample of each item.

Place a large scoop or serving spoon in each bowl. Include a second smaller spoon, about the size of a typical teaspoon that we use to stir our tea or coffee. The two options allow toddlers to make a choice and encourage any hesitant eater at the table to have just a sample on their plate. As the master server plates each person's dinner per their request, they get repeated exposure to the foods. Each plate is then passed back to the family member, and another person passes their plate up to the master server. This technique is especially helpful for toddlers in the natural phase of picky eating. Learning to become an adventurous eater is always about repeated exposures, even if it's simply spooning a tiny bit of new food onto our plate.

> ## "In our family, we have a bit of everything on our plate."
>
> For typically developing toddlers and older children, establish a rule early on that we always have a bit of everything on our plate. Notice how I didn't say "a bite" of

everything? When raising children in a responsive feeding household, kids are willing to take a bite because they listen to their internal body cues and desire to eat or not eat. The catalyst for taking a bite is simply the exposure to small samples on the plate. There's no need to command a bite. In fact, research shows that for our garden-variety picky eaters, those extra bites won't help kids grow if they are underweight nor will it change their behavior. All it really does is ease the parent's own anxiety based on their own expectations of what they think their child should eat.[3]

Pre-Plating Strategies

Small samples are a key element when pre-plating for toddlers and hesitant eaters. In earlier chapters, I shared a basic guideline on portion sizes for mealtimes equivalent to one tablespoon per year of age. If you're certain that your toddler is not likely to try a new food, reducing the sample to just one teaspoon is certainly fine, and it reduces food waste. If at least one familiar food is offered, your toddler will have plenty to fill their belly. For familiar foods, stick to the "one tablespoon per year of age" rule and allow for more when that portion is consumed.

Eat this, then that

Eating one food should never be contingent upon getting more of a preferred food. "Eat two peas and then you can have more mac-n-cheese" is never a strategy that aligns with responsive feeding practices. Does it really matter if a toddler doesn't eat a few peas tonight? No. Peace at mealtimes is always more important than peas at mealtimes.

There are pros and cons to family-style versus pre-plating, but one is not better than the other. Each child is different, and each family is different. My advice? Do both. Family-style requires a bit more prep and may help anxious eaters learn to tolerate new foods on the table, and eventually on their plate. There is an art to pre-plating. Make each portion small, so it's not overwhelming. Everyone gets the same foods on their plate. If kids protest, treat the food like a tiny sprig of decorative parsley on the plate. It's just there. "Yep, honey, we all have parsley (broccoli, green beans, and so on) on our plates." Then move on. There is no more discussion about the food—take the attention off it.

Sugar & Artificial Sweeteners: Restrict or Regulate?

If your child has not shown an interest in sugar by age two, there isn't any urgency to introduce them to it. However, children with different food personalities can and will coexist in the same family and social circles, so parents need to consider a strategy toward sweets that promotes the child's self-regulation (rather than a sense of restriction).

Ashley Smith, an RDN from veggiesandvirtue.com, suggests that parents consider the role sugar plays in their child's overall diet and development, and approach it more intentionally, instead of with fear-based approaches. Ashley explained as follows:

ADVICE FROM AN EXPERT NUTRITIONIST

Nutritionally speaking, most young children who eat a variety of foods do not "need" added sugar in their diet because they consume naturally occurring sugar from grains, fruits, and vegetables. Usually by age two, children begin to be aware of and express more interest in sweets, both inside and outside the home. These might include those with nonnutritive sweeteners (such as aspartame, sucralose, and stevia, among others), sugar alcohols (which you can identify on an ingredient list as those ending in -ol), and sugar (in the more obvious forms of cane sugar, brown sugar, honey, fructose, or maple syrup, and so on). If not careful, parents can misunderstand which of these is "best" to include in their child's diet, especially when the emphasis with sugar often seems to be to eat "less."

Nonnutritive sweeteners (NNS) are often used in attempts to decrease overall sugar intake and lower caloric intake from sugar-sweetened foods like soda, sports drinks, and candy. Another form of "sugar-free" sugar are sugar alcohols. Like NNSs, these are generally recognized as safe to consume and can appeal to parents because such sweeteners allow food to be marketed as sugar free or reduced sugar, and yet provide a sweetness kids crave. However, the research on NNSs in toddlers and children remains limited. We know that NNSs provide a sweet taste ranging from 180 to 20,000 times sweeter than traditional table sugar and may be associated with greater preference for sweet foods in children.[4] Even in at-risk populations (e.g., children with diabetes or obesity), recommendations for the use or avoidance of NNSs remain conflicting because the impact on body weight, insulin resistance, and long-term metabolic risk are unknown.

With this, NNSs are not at all the obvious solution to satisfying a child's normal, natural sugar craving—and especially not early on. Instead, families ought to adopt dessert policies that allow for regular access to and inclusion of sugar. Structuring meals, snacks, and celebrations where sugar will be offered provides children with critical opportunities to become more relaxed and better able to self-regulate their sugar intake. As with best practices for feeding other foods, parents get to decide what, when, and where such sweets and treats are offered. Their child then gets to decide whether and how much they want to eat. Including regular sweets allows children to satisfy their cravings while still ensuring that their nutritional needs are being met with the more nutrient-dense foods that make up most of their diet. Finding this balance will be unique to each family and child, but when parents put the emphasis on mindfully enjoying sweet foods with their children from early on, they are likely to raise a child who innately understands how all foods fit together for a healthy diet and proper development.

> ## Take dessert off the pedestal
> ## (or never put it there in the first place)
>
> A small cookie, a scatter of mini chocolate chips, or a tiny scoop of sorbet is a fun addition to the dinner plate without making dessert the endgame for mealtime. When a small sampling of sweets is just part of the meal or snack, kids learn to enjoy all kinds of food without making one food the ultimate treat. Fresh asparagus straight from the garden is a treat, too! It's all in how you frame it. You may be wondering what to do if you have a child under the age of two as well as older kids, given the "no added sugar" rule for younger children. Be strategic and offer sweets after the younger child has gone to bed or provide a lower-sugar alternative on both of their plates. For example, try offering "three-ingredient cookies" made from bananas, oatmeal, and just a few mini chocolate chips sprinkled on top. It's a popular recipe found on the internet that's quick and easy—and freezes well, too!

Fun Ways to Encourage Toddlers to Drink Water

According to the Harvard T.H. Chan School of Public Health, "more than half of all children and adolescents in the U.S. are not getting enough hydration—probably because they're not drinking enough water—a situation that could have significant repercussions for their physical health and their cognitive and emotional functioning."[5] Drinking water is essential for both body and brain health, and even mild dehydration causes reduced cognitive functioning. Kids can't learn if they aren't hydrated, and it will be reflected in their mood and energy levels, too.[6] Foster a love for water by incorporating a bit of fun and making it easy for your child. Here are five tips to encourage toddlers to drink more water:

1. **Tiny bears:** Kids love anything tiny and cute, and what's cuter than an itty-bitty bear with a straw for those big, little, and "just-right" sips? Whether your toddler is a fan of Goldilocks and the Three Bears or not, the six-ounce bears designed for small containers of honey are perfect to foster a love for water. The size is ideal for a toddler-size grasp and the ideal height when placed on the table for a smaller child. Simply insert a silicone straw into the top (where the honey squirts out) and kids cannot resist taking a sip! With such a small cup, it's much easier for kids to "drink it all gone" and be ready to refill it throughout the day. Tip: Fill the cup halfway if your toddler discovers that a strong squeeze on the bear's full belly will make water squirt across the table! Both silicone straws and small honey bears are found on Amazon.com.

2. **Homemade aquarium:** One of my favorite strategies for encouraging kids to refill their cups involves filling a spouted water container and creating an incentive to visit it often. First, position the container at the back of the countertop, where kids cannot pull it over onto the floor. Place a few heavy books under the container to raise the spout up so a small cup fits underneath. Every time the child finishes their cup of water, say, "Let's go add another sea creature to the ocean!" Keep a stash of clean plastic sharks, dolphins, and fun sea creatures for the child to pick from and add to the "ocean." It's the perfect motivation to visit several times a day, but an empty cup is required to do so. The kids don't get to play with the sea animals at any other time—this keeps it novel for frequent requests to visit their aquarium!

3. **Cup fairy house:** Help kids make a cardboard house for the "cup fairy," who brings a new cup every morning just for them! Buy inexpensive cups with lids and straws and let your

child add their favorite stickers to each new cup that appears each day. Say, "Let's see what the cup fairy brought for you!" Then take your toddler to the cup house and let them pull out a brand-new cup. Now, go the homemade aquarium (see #2 above) and fill it up! The next day, a new cup will appear. It takes about two weeks for toddlers to get into the habit of drinking more water, and this is an inexpensive way to get them excited to see what the cup fairy brought that morning.

4. **Infused water:** Adding fruits, herbs, and vegetables to create subtly flavored water is an excellent way to get kids involved in handling new foods, encourage them to drink more water, and perhaps try a new food, too! Using kid-safe knives, help toddlers slice cucumbers, mint, watermelon, and other foods to add to the water. Popular combinations include oranges and strawberries, cucumbers and mint, pomegranate seeds and cantaloupe.

5. **Model good habits:** Kids learn best through modeling, so grab your own water bottle and enjoy![7]

Be polite and kind at mealtimes

By age three, establish basic rules for mealtimes in and out of the home:

- If you don't have a nice thing to say about the food, don't say anything at all. Don't yuck somebody else's yum!

- We smile and say thank you when served food, even if we decide not to eat it.

- You don't have to eat, but you do need to sit and socialize at the table. This is a special time—it's family time.

- At home, we always take our plate to the counter when we are done.

The Research Supporting
Family Mealtimes

Family Meals Help You Raise Healthier Kids

Just three family mealtimes per week has been shown to positively influence the nutritional health of toddlers to adolescents. In fact, in a meta-analysis of seventeen different studies, the results were clear: Children are less likely to be overweight and eat unhealthy foods, and they're 35 percent less likely to develop disordered eating than kids who do not have regular family mealtimes.[8] Healthy bodies also mean healthier minds. Family meals strongly impact a child's preschool, primary, and secondary school performance, as well as their emotional and mental health.

Family Meals Help You Raise Smarter Kids

Family mealtime provides consistent opportunities to reconnect in our busy lives, share values and ideas, and parent mindfully. Need a little motivation to make family mealtime a regular habit? Your kid will be smarter because of it. Research demonstrates that routine family meals play a crucial role in language development in young children.[9] I've previously written that "both expressive and receptive language skills improve when children are a part of the mealtime table with their parents and older siblings, and those mealtime conversations also seem to influence early reading skills, as measured by improvement in reading scores."[10]

Reading is always a good thing, but here's a startling fact: Researchers found that for young children, dinnertime conversation trumps even story time![11] When you read aloud to your children, it supports language and literacy development, including exposing your child to atypical vocabulary or those words not used in common day-to-day interactions. But during dinnertime conversation, young children learn 1,000 rare words! That in turn supports reading development, and those children learn to read earlier than their peers.[12]

The kind of conversation around the table helps raise smarter kids, too! Think about it . . . what did you talk about last night at dinner? Most likely, you conveyed information via storytelling. You may have told your partner what your toddler did at the park that day or the unexpected sequence of events when they discovered a mud puddle! Mealtime conversation is most often conveyed via storytelling or narratives. Soon, when your toddler enters preschool, they will be at a distinct advantage that will last into their teen years. Preschoolers who have strong storytelling skills now, have higher reading scores in high school![13]

Family Meals Help You Raise Safer Kids

The benefits of consistent family meals, just three to five per week, are evident for our young children. Older children reap the academic benefits as well. Adolescents who have family meals at least five times per week were twice as likely to get As in school than kids who only ate dinner with their families two times per week.[14] The advantages don't stop there. The kids in the first group also made safer decisions around life choices. Research from Columbia University has shown that the benefits continue for a lifetime. Teens who have three or more meals with their family each week have a decreased risk of drug, alcohol, and cigarette use, and more.

Family Meals Decrease Family Stress

By raising a child in a responsive feeding household, you are setting the stage for joyful and stress-free mealtimes. Staying warm and engaged, the essence of responsive feeding, can be challenging at times, given a toddler's strong opinions and emotions. Rest assured that, armed with the strategies discussed in this chapter, the majority of meals at your table will go smoothly. Studies show that evening meals together, even though most last for just twenty minutes, improve the moods of older children and adults who have had a stressful day. Family dinner is a time to decompress and connect, and is simply good for the soul.

Dr. Anne Fischel of Harvard Medical School—an expert in the research behind family mealtimes at The Family Dinner Project (thefamilydinnerproject.org)—counsels parents that "as long as there are two family members eating together, experiencing connection, and enjoying one another, that is a family dinner. The adult could be an aunt, grandfather, or another caregiver."[15]

Everyone in the family benefits from regular family meals, whether it be breakfast, a picnic at the park, or simply a parent sitting with a cup of tea while your toddler is having lunch beside you. It's not the table where you sit, it's who is sitting at the table that's most important.

Chapter Six

Eating Away from Home & Navigating Family Influences

Wherever you are on your journey, from the first introduction of solids to the first day of preschool, be prepared for other people to express their opinion on exactly how you should feed your child. Most suggestions from outside influences (teachers, relatives, friends) are meant to be helpful, although they can feel more like a roadblock to the beautiful feeding relationship you've created with your child. Rather than seeing them as obstacles, think of these moments as road signs that may indicate how to remain on the path to responsive feeding (or not).

Responding to Strong Opinions from the People You Love

Dani Lebovitz—the author of *101 Descriptive Words for Food Explorers*, one of my favorite books on building your child's food vocabulary—is an RD with a wealth of knowledge regarding one of the most challenging issues for new parents: how to respond to everyone else's strong opinions about how to feed YOUR baby. These often come from the people you love, including your own mom, your grandparents, or your spouse's family. As Dani and I chatted about this dilemma, she offered the following advice for parents introducing responsive feeding practices to well-meaning adults who offer their own advice on how to feed your kid.[1]

ADVICE FROM AN EXPERT DIETITIAN

Family dynamics play a key role in the way we feed children, as values, attitudes, and beliefs are often passed from one generation to the next. Additional factors that influence a person's unique feeding beliefs include cultural background, personal experience, and economic environment. As a result, sometimes there are disagreements on feeding practices between parents, and often grandparents, who have recommendations for how to feed children based on how they were raised and how they raised their children. This is especially true when feeding practices are passed down from generation to generation. Well-meaning family members may assert that their feeding approach is the "correct" method, which disparages the wishes of parents, especially new parents.[2]

Breaking this cycle can be a challenge as parents work to feed their child the way they want to feed them and create positive associations around mealtime in the manner of responsive feeding practices.

Here are three tools to navigate these challenging conversations:

1. **Try to understand family history**

   The first step to developing a supportive feeding environment in your home is to learn about each partner's mealtime and feeding practices that they experienced in their households growing up. Discuss what meals were like from a cultural standpoint, rules around meals, and how food scarcity or abundance of food changed mealtime.

   Having these conversations is important to understanding how ingrained certain feeding practices are and help put them in perspective. Not only will this help you empathize with each other's feeding beliefs, but it will also help you understand your own values and approach.

2. **Discuss your feeding approach as a family and develop a plan**

   After understanding each other's background and feeding influences, it's time to develop a united approach to feeding your child. Take some time to talk about what is important and find ways to meet in the middle, supporting the values and beliefs of each partner.

   If there are inconsistencies between thoughts or desires and actions, then talk about them. Sometimes a neutral third party can be a helpful mediator. Remember, you share the same goal: raising a healthy child who has a healthy relationship with food.

3. **Discuss your feeding approach with family members**

   Recognize that family members may not agree or support your approach to feeding your child, and that is OK. When discussing your feeding approach with well-meaning family members, start by identifying their positive suggestions that you plan to incorporate and what you like about them. This helps family members feel heard and acknowledged. Then, share your desired approach while noting that feeding practices change over time and this is what you want for your family. Keep the focus on the well-being of your child and that you and your partner decide the rules for your family.

Here are some helpful prompts to use with well-meaning family members:

- "Watching for _____'s hunger and fullness cues is very important to us to create a positive feeding experience. Here are some cues you may notice . . ." Then share their signs of hunger and fullness.

- "We follow the belief that 'we provide and _____ decides.' This sets them up for healthy growth and development."

- "We have done a lot of research on how we want to feed _____. Please support us on this, even if you don't agree."

- "We feel really strongly about not forcing _____ to finish their meal. Please support us on this, even if you don't agree."

Infusing the Flavors of Your Heritage

Infusing the flavors of your heritage can be delicate if your child is a bit hesitant or has special needs. Sophia Hazan, a speech pathologist and feeding specialist in New York City, lives in a community where traditional culture and a history of flavors and fellowship play a key role in how children are fed. I asked Sophia to share her experiences as both a member of her community and as a professional who shares the joy of responsive feeding practices with her clients. Sophia explains[3]:

ADVICE FROM AN EXPERT FEEDING SPECIALIST

To many people, culture, tradition, and religion play an essential role in what, when, how, and why their families eat. The importance of each dish often comes from ancient religious practices, and historic events or circumstances. When it comes to feeding children, parents and grandparents of these rich historical cultures want nothing more than to pass on these significant recipes that have lived on for hundreds of years, and to see their offspring enjoy them. An example of a tight-knit and religious community who held on to its culinary treasures and intriguing customs is the Sephardic Orthodox Jewish community. The Sephardic Jews mark religious events, holidays, and life-cycle events by celebrating with traditional meals and customary dishes.

Fleeing Spain after being expelled in 1492, the Jews found refuge in Middle Eastern countries such as Turkey, Syria, and Egypt. Over the course of hundreds of years, these Jews cultivated their own cuisine by combining theirs with the flavors, cooking styles, spices, and herbs of their neighbors. Hospitality was a foundational part of their religion, and their doors were always open to others

When the Jews of Aleppo, Syria, immigrated to America in the early twentieth century, their rich cuisine and spirited culture came with them. During these assimilation years, maintaining their Syrian-Jewish recipes was more important to them than ever before. Food was often scarce for fresh immigrants, and families with many children found themselves rationing their meals. I remember my own grandfather, who was the youngest of ten children, used to say, "If I didn't eat quick, I didn't eat at all." Furthermore, many immigrants arrived in America just prior to the Great Depression and were all too familiar with bread lines, food rations, and shortages. The members of that generation appreciated food in a way their grandchildren and great-grandchildren could not.

When treating babies and children in my own Syrian-Jewish community, it came as no surprise that parents and grandparents alike have a strong passion for maintaining their food culture. They want their babies to enjoy the same food experiences that they had growing up. Oftentimes, family members from older generations do not understand the issues that children with pediatric feeding disorders face. They may even express their concerns or have questions regarding the methodology feeding therapists use with these extreme "picky eaters." As a feeding therapist, I know it is important to provide evidence-based practices while simultaneously respecting the family and their unique food culture. Being sensitive to these cultural differences is essential to working with any child. Asking about the family's food culture and traditions at the commencement of therapy is helpful. Understanding the family dynamic, as well as their expectations regarding food goals, food prep, etiquette, and dietary restrictions, is also an important consideration. My ultimate goal as a feeding therapist is to be conscious of all of these considerations and tailor a successful therapy program that is appropriate for each individual child and their family.

> ## Creating community support
>
> Our close-knit communities, such as places of worship and preschool, genuinely want to be supportive of children with special needs, including those with allergies and medical conditions. Offer to present a short informational talk at a community function or ask a professional to help present the information. Whenever I volunteer to educate, the communities have always been welcoming! The most common feedback I receive is "I had no idea! Thank you for sharing that with us!" The more they know, the more they want to help.

Day Care & Preschool

If you're considering sending your young child to day care or preschool, it may feel unsettling to trust in the foundation of responsive feeding that you have created at home. Ten years ago, Dr. Nimali Fernando (aka Dr. Yum) and I created the Doctor Yum Preschool Food Adventure, an evidence-based, interactive curriculum designed to encourage a responsive feeding model while incorporating sensory activities to foster the joy of eating fruits and vegetables. We trained preschool teachers to read and respect the child's cues and gently guide them to explore new foods. One of those very first preschool teachers, Wendy Cannon, was the director of a Virginia preschool and has over 20 years of experience. To help you explore options for your child's care and food education that will support the responsive feeding paradigm, Ms. Cannon, an expert preschool teacher, offered the following advice[4]:

When researching childcare and preschool programs, ask about their food policies. The director should be able to share a written copy with you. Food policies may also include information about whether the school provides the meals/snacks or if the students bring their own. Confirm that there are policies in place for:

- Foods that are considered choking hazards
- Foods that are not allowed due to allergies
- Consideration for the individual student's food restrictions/preferences (including but not limited to vegetarian, vegan, kosher or halal)
- Nutritional expectations for food brought in by students
- Foods brought in by students that don't meet the food policies
- Not using food as a reward or punishment
- Birthday or holiday celebrations

It is also important to ask what mealtimes are like in the program:

- Do students and teachers sit down to eat together?
- Are there expectations for what foods and how much students are supposed to eat?
- Are children allowed additional helpings if they are still hungry?
- Are children allowed to determine when they are done eating?

Teachers should be accepting of each child's own barometer for what and how much they eat at a particular meal or snack time. Children are much more in tune with their own hunger and fullness cues than adults give them credit for!

A child should never be forced to taste or take a bite of a particular food. Many foods are new experiences for preschoolers, and they may need multiple sensory exposures to a particular food before they are ready to taste. Instead, children are encouraged to be "food explorers," which allows them opportunities to become friends with new foods and reduces anxiety around new food experiences.

Write a note

Selective eaters may feel more pressure to eat outside the home environment if they are unsure of expectations or if the rules are very strict. A note that outlines responsive feeding practices from their feeding therapist in their file at school is helpful, but the substitute teachers and supporting lunch staff may not see it or remember the details. Some parents choose to put a card in the lunchbox explaining their child's eating style. Others prefer to have several printed and kept in the child's cubby or backpack. Choose whatever location will ensure that the card will be seen. A sample card might read:

Dear _____,

In our household, we are practicing responsive feeding with (child's name), and we follow one hard-and-fast rule to help him eat. It's pretty simple—just let him eat and/or drink whatever he wants in his lunchbox and don't comment on it. If he doesn't eat anything, he'll be OK. If that happens, would you please quietly let me know? There are things that I can do here at home to help him feel confident in his eating at (day care, school) and we can chat about those another time. Thank you for supporting us! I'm available anytime if you have questions at _____.

Warmly,

(Your name)

At Ms. Cannon's cooperative preschool, the snack each day is brought in by a student known as the "special helper" and their "helper parent." One year, a student loved sugar snap peas and brought them, along with cheese and crackers, for the class snack. A few classmates were familiar with sugar snap peas, but many were not. Each student had two sugar snap peapods on their plate. Some popped them open to count the peas inside, some took a practice bite, and others did not try them at all. This parent decided that she would bring sugar snap peas as part of their snack for the rest of the year. So about once a month, these students all got another exposure to two sugar snap peapods on their plates, and it was amazing to see more and more kids trying them as the year went on! Exposure is everything. This is a great example of putting responsive feeding into practice.

Packed lunches

When sending your little one off to day care with a packed lunch, set them up for success with an easy-open lunchbox and minimal packaging. Shallow bento boxes are ideal; just be sure the latch is easily opened by little hands and kids can comfortably view what's inside. It's difficult for small children to peer inside a deep bento box on a tall table. Extra packaging, like bags of crackers or wrapping on cheese, is unnecessary and time-consuming for littles to attempt to open. Be sure that all the food is chopped into safe, manageable pieces, and include a small ice pack on top of the bento box to ensure that the foods stay fresh. Tape a fork or spoon to the top of the box if there is not a compartment inside for utensil storage. To ensure that kids have time to fill their bellies and still enjoy some social time with friends, try what I call "grab and gab food." Pack the lunch box with easy-to-grab fruit chunks, blanched and cooled vegetables, and perhaps a protein like moist pieces of chicken. When children have a smorgasbord of options, they can reach in, grab a piece, and still gab (even in toddler language!) with their friends.

Hot items should be opened only by a teacher. When sending a thermos or container that keeps foods like macaroni and cheese warm, store the container in a separate area in your child's backpack. Include a note on the bento box that reads, "Warm mac 'n' cheese in the outer pocket of backpack for teacher to open!" to alert an adult.

Use lunch packing as a way to continue to expose your child to foods that they are still learning to appreciate. Pack several preferred foods and include about a teaspoon of a food that your child isn't so keen about. If your child goes to day care just three times per week, that's over 150 opportunities in a year to expose them to small samples of those foods. Exposure is everything, so don't miss your chance to expand your child's palate! If that bit of food comes back home uneaten, that's never a waste. It's just the first step to eventually tasting it.

Restaurants

Four words: Skip the kids' menu. You've worked diligently to raise your child to love a variety of foods, often the exact same foods that you're eating, too. Since you've raised the bar on your child's culinary preferences, why order from a mini menu that sets the bar very, very low? It's tempting because the kids' menu appears to have smaller portions for a lower price than the adult menu. Guess what's even less expensive with more culinary exposure? Small samples of whatever you're ordering.

Ask the waiter for an extra plate or simply bring your favorite stick-to-the-table plate for your little one. You are now well versed in how to safely cut and serve many different foods, and you'll be following the same strategies when dining at restaurants and other outings. Order an extra side dish if needed. Even if you're ordering a salad at the local drive-thru or fast-food restaurant, consider skipping the kids' meal and creating a kid's sampling of grilled chicken cubes, shredded carrots, chopped mandarin oranges, or other options directly from your salad when you arrive at your destination. Request an extra packet of dressing if your kid likes to dip.

Feeding Myths that
Impact Development

The toddler years can be challenging in a variety of ways, and it's easy for others to brush off concerns you have about your child's eating patterns. You may be hearing reassurance from well-meaning friends and family, like "All toddlers are picky! Eventually they grow out of it" and "Relax! No kid ever starved because he only ate chicken nuggets." In the next chapter, I'll share information about the importance of early intervention when a child's feeding development seems to stall. Here are some of the common feeding myths that often prevent a child from getting the help they need early in life:

All toddlers are picky! They will grow out of it.

This is the most common myth of all. Dr. Mitchell Katz, director of the Multidisciplinary Feeding Program at the Children's Hospital of California (who also wrote the foreword for this book) recently sat down with me for an interview. He told me that the most important advocate for the child is the parent. But the parent must feel heard. If the parent is seeing that their child is not progressing in development, they have the right not to be told, "Oh don't worry about it, they'll outgrow it." It may be that simple interventions might be needed before the issue becomes a bigger one. Why wait? Dr. Katz says, "The earlier you get to a problem, the easier it is to solve."

In the next chapter, you'll learn what signs may indicate the need for early intervention and how to discuss your concerns with your pediatrician to ensure that your child gets the support they need to create happier mealtimes.

Kids don't need to use utensils! Let them use their hands!

Feeding is developmental and includes the interplay between gross-motor and fine-motor skills. Fine-motor skills include self-feeding, the pincer grasp, and utensil use, as well as age-appropriate chewing and swallowing—and these skills set your three-year-old kid up for other developments that they will need in preschool. By age three, kids' fine-motor skills allow them to button and unbutton, build a tower of ten blocks, complete puzzles of more than five pieces, and manipulate pencils and crayons. They can make a circle with a crayon on a piece of paper, cut the paper with child-safe scissors, and string large beads. If you have any concerns about your child's fine-motor development, bring it to your pediatrician's attention. They may recommend a free or low-cost evaluation through your local school district or with a licensed pediatric occupational therapist in your community.

My toddler's frequent coughing is a normal way to protect their airway.

Speech pathologists who specialize in pediatric swallowing disorders often say that a good cough is good to hear! A cough is a protective reflex that protects a child's airway by clearing debris from the throat, larynx (voice box), and trachea (windpipe) so that food or objects don't enter the lungs. Some children don't have a strong reflex and will aspirate food easily because their brain doesn't sense the need to cough. So when SLPs hear that a child coughed and expelled the offending debris, that means the safety mechanism is working. However, too much coughing can indicate that your child is having trouble coordinating the muscles and mechanics of swallowing. If you've ever had a bit of water or food "go down the wrong pipe" and suddenly started coughing, you know how uncomfortable that feeling can be. Repeated coughing is not pleasant, and it creates a negative association with mealtimes and sometimes with specific foods. Coughing a lot may also indicate aspiration, and that can lead to serious respiratory issues.

If your toddler coughs on occasion when eating, perhaps a few times a week, it's likely a good thing. But if they are coughing daily or frequently enough that you are wondering about this behavior, be sure to tell your pediatrician. There are simple tests that can help SLPs and other medical professionals visualize what's happening when your child swallows. These preliminary tests will help rule out medical challenges that could lead to more serious health issues in the future.

He's extremely picky, but he's following his curve, so it's fine.

As mentioned in the section on growth and appetite (see page 120), the growth curve tells a story. There's much more to a child's feeding journey than plotting a curve. If picky eating at mealtimes is causing stress in your family, that is the number one reason to insist on a pediatric feeding evaluation. Learning to eat is a complex process! Following a responsive feeding model is considered best practice, but feeding is still a developmental process. So if your child is stalling in development, it's time to seek help.

Chapter Seven

Red Flags & Special Needs

Before becoming a speech pathologist and working with children with special needs, I was raising my own two children, one an adventurous eater and one a more hesitant eater. That's when I started to put the pieces together that would eventually spark my interest in responsive feeding practices. I didn't parent my eager eater any differently than my hesitant eater, but there she was, becoming pickier every day. The reason? Her oral sensory system for flavors and texture was quite different from her sister's, and trying new food was more challenging.

At the time, I didn't know how to express my concerns to my pediatrician. Everyone told me that "all kids are picky" and "no kid will starve." Sadly, now that I've made it my profession, I know that those statements diminish a parent's concern. The other issue for families with apprehensive eaters is the stress it can bring to *everyone* in the household. Fortunately, I took a breath and considered what was most important at mealtimes—my family. I focused on our time together and exposing both kids to a variety of foods. Sure, some days my toddlers had fish crackers and a juice box for snack but on most days, I offered more balanced variety at meals and snacks. Helping a child become an adventurous eater takes time and conscious effort from parents, but you don't have to do it on your own when you know how to ask for help.

One out of four typically developing children will develop a feeding disorder that can impact growth, nutritional health, and family and peer relationships. Rather than worrying about your child's fussy eating, learn specific strategies from an expert that you can implement at home. Often an evaluation with a few suggestions from a therapist is all you will need, and at other times children can attend weekly sessions to find the joy in food. It's well worth the time to learn how to help when you consider the daily impact of frustrating and stressful breakfasts, lunches, dinners, and snacks.

Pausing to Chat with Your Pediatrician

Time is scarce when visiting your pediatrician. Constraints due to insurance criteria and other demands on their time result in a highly regimented schedule. It's a heavy burden for most primary care physicians when they are forced to reduce the minutes they can spend with each family. The median length of a visit to a primary care physician's office is 15.7 minutes, covering six different topics![1] Pediatricians genuinely want to spend more time counseling parents and caregivers, answering their questions, and collaborating as a team for the best care for each child.

If you have concerns about your child's feeding development, and even if a well-child visit is scheduled in the very near future, there may be a few minutes to list the red flags you're encountering at home. Consider scheduling a special visit to dive deeper into the issue so that your child's physician has a clear understanding and can schedule appropriate referrals immediately. For children under the age of three, early intervention has proved to be the best course of action. The Centers for Disease Control and Prevention (CDC) recommends calling your state or territory's early intervention program to request an assessment.* A doctor's referral is not necessary, but pausing to discuss your concerns with your pediatrician creates a team of support for both you and your child.

Early intervention provides speech therapy, physical therapy, occupational therapy, and other services for children up to age three who have developmental delays or disabilities. Remember, feeding is a developmental process. Delays in feeding development can cause children to be underweight or represent a failure to thrive, impacting brain growth. Feeding challenges can be incredibly stressful for the entire family, and it's best not to wait for children to "grow out of it." In fact, 1 out of 4 children do not grow out of hesitant eating and will receive the diagnosis of a pediatric feeding disorder. It's not unusual for kids to have difficulty eating, and you are not alone. Recent research has found that up to 50 percent of "normally developing children are reported to experience some type of feeding problem."[2]

Your pediatrician is the first source of information about local hospitals and private clinics that provide feeding therapy. SLPs and OTs who specialize in pediatric feeding work in a variety of settings, often making home visits or working on a feeding team in a medical setting. Talk to your pediatrician about the best environment to fit the needs of you and your child. This may depend on the signs and symptoms of feeding distress and whether medical testing is the first course of action. The earlier you note the red flags,

---

* Your pediatrician or primary care doctor can provide phone numbers for your state's early intervention program, or visit cdc.gov/ncbddd/actearly/parents/states.html for specific information for your area.

the sooner your little one will receive an assessment and possible intervention, leading to happier mealtimes for all in the future.

Red flags

The number one reason to consult with your pediatrician about a feeding assessment is because feeding your child is not an enjoyable experience and it causes stress for you, your partner, your other children, and/or your hesitant eater. Here are some of the red flags indicating a possible feeding disorder:

- Your child is not gaining weight.

- Your child is not transitioning from breastfeeding or bottle-feeding to solids on an appropriate developmental timeline.

- Your child vomits daily or is distressed by frequent gagging.

- Your child coughs frequently during or after mealtimes.

- Your child is not able to drink from a straw or an open cup, or use utensils on an appropriate developmental timeline.

- Your child's behavior at mealtimes is distressing. For example, they refuse to sit in their high chair, repeatedly spit out food and demand milk, or have emotional outbursts on a regular basis.

- Your child eats well at day care or for others, but not at home.

- Your child eats well at home, but not at day care or for other caregivers.

- Your child has a limited repertoire of foods that they will eat. The options may be restricted to certain brands, or a short list of favorite foods or food textures.

Tips for Communicating with Your Child's Pediatrician

A pediatrician's job is to help kids grow and learn, monitoring their health and development along the way to ensure that even a minor stall in development doesn't lead to bigger issues. While it may be tempting just to give your child more time to develop certain skills, it can have detrimental consequences if it causes a delay in physical, cognitive, or emotional growth. To ensure that you express your concerns clearly and concisely during the time you have in their doctor's office, come prepared. Here are three tips to optimize the time and get the results you need for your little one:

1. Leave distractions at home. Whenever possible, find a babysitter to watch your other children and bring only the hesitant eater to the appointment. It sounds simple, but please remember to silence your phone so that text messages and phone calls aren't distracting for you or your doctor.

2. Use your phone to convey the truth. Take pictures of your child's breakfast, lunch, dinner, and snack plates before they begin eating and after they are done over the course of one day. Providing a visual of what was served, how much was consumed, and at what time of day provides concrete information in an efficient manner. Video a mealtime to share segments of behaviors that you find stressful and difficult to manage.

3. Have a script ready and rehearsed. Know exactly what you plan to say and, most important, know what you want to accomplish in the conversation. If the goal is to get a feeding evaluation for your child, state that in clear, concise language:

   - **State your concern:** "I am concerned that feeding my child is so stressful. There's no joy in our mealtimes."
   - **Show the proof:** "I've brought you some pictures and a short video to show you what has been happening at home."
   - **Tell them what you need:** "I'd like to discuss getting a feeding evaluation for my child."

Child Feeding Questionnaire

Feedingmatters.org has an evidence-based tool to help parents with early identification of possible feeding disorders in their children from birth to age three. Visit their website to fill in the digital questionnaire and learn more.

There are seven Cs to effective communication[3] with your child's physician.

1. Be Clear. What is your main message?

2. Be Concise. Don't waste time.

3. Be Concrete. Stick to the script.

4. Be Correct. Make sure the facts are correct, especially if you are relaying another person's input, like your speech pathologist's findings.

5. Be Courteous. Your child's doctor wants to help.

6. Be Curious. Be open to options that may be presented in the meeting.

7. Call to Action: Once you've followed the six Cs above and considered everyone's opinions, state exactly what you need before the appointment ends.

Feeding a Medically Complex Child in a Responsive Way

Because feeding is a developmental journey, challenges can arise for a variety of reasons. Kids typically learn to avoid certain foods, becoming more rigid over time, if they experience repeated discomfort from a physical or emotional standpoint.

Picture three blocks, stacked on top of each other. The first block is physiology, and it's the foundation for learning how to eat. When something goes awry with a child's physiology, it means the body or brain isn't functioning the way it should. It might be due to a clear physiological difference, like a cleft palate, or the issue might be more hidden, like an overactive sensory system. (These are just two examples; there are hundreds more!) Physiology also includes brain functioning where anxiety, temperament, learning, and attention issues all come into play. The second block consists of gross- and fine-motor skills. Fine-motor stability is always dependent on how well a child's gross-motor skills develop, and these in turn can impact feeding skills. The third block is learned behaviors. Picky eaters, mild to extreme, behave the way they do around food because they are protecting themselves. They learn very quickly that eating hurts, either physically or emotionally. In fact, in the first four weeks of life, a baby will learn to turn away from the bottle if eating is uncomfortable. Research continues to show that positive early experiences with food are critical to raising healthy, happy eaters.

Feeding disorders are not limited to children with special needs. Approximately 25 percent of normally developing children experience feeding problems.[4] Whether or not the child has physiological or motor issues, a primary focus of all feeding therapy needs to be the transactional nature of the parent–child relationship. That is the essence of responsive feeding.

A study in the Journal of Pediatric Psychology examined the parent–child relationship in children with feeding disorders (FDs) who did not present with organic or medical conditions that could explain their feeding difficulties and had no developmental delays. The findings emphasized that "interventions tailored to families with a child with a [FD] should focus on mealtime dynamics. A better understanding of their children's behaviors and needs (e.g., desire for independence, including autonomy in eating), and assistance in identifying strategies to avoid mealtime battles may be particularly helpful."[5]

With the right feeding therapy, therapists help kids "unlearn" these behaviors, replacing the undesired behaviors (avoiding new food experiences and environments, turning away from the spoon, spitting food, and so on) with positive interactions that foster a joy for all kinds of delicious foods. In my entire career, I've never met a child who had developed a behavioral feeding problem just for the heck of it. Kids communicate via behavior, and it takes an experienced and compassionate feeding specialist to be that child's personal detective to solve all the pieces of the puzzle. The behaviors are just what we see. Our job is to discover the reasons behind the behavior.

The methods for helping a child embrace the joy of food vary, because no two children are alike. But when using a step-by-step, compassionate methodology, the best therapists guide not just the child, but the entire family to developing a responsive feeding framework. In my own work with extreme picky eaters, my goal is to boost the child's skill, trust, and confidence in their own abilities and then guide the entire family to embrace responsive feeding practice.

There are many evidence-based methods to help children learn to eat a variety of tastes and textures and embrace the joy for food. In feeding therapy, some therapists may utilize the principles of responsive feeding from the very start. Other therapists may incorporate more of a hybrid approach. This is where experience and evidence-based practice are crucial to determine what strategies work best for each family. Ultimately the goal is to settle into the model of responsive feeding before discharging the child from therapy. Feeding therapy is a bit like riding a bike, but first we need some training wheels before we learn to glide along on our own.

Gentle Pushes

There is an art to building skill and ability, and then supporting via gentle pushes to help kids take the next step in their feeding journey. Like any compassionate athletic coach, feeding therapists recognize that eating isn't a skill that comes easily to some kids. Even when therapists address medical, motor, sensory, or other factors that influence a child's ability to taste a new food, the anxiety is often still present for kids of any age. Even after consistent therapeutic support, these children tend to stick to their safe foods, no matter what. It can be scary to step outside that safe zone! In these situations, kids may require more direct instructions from the therapist to lead them to a new safe place. Think of feeding therapy as gentle guidance, using light, fingertip nudges to help kids inch outside their safe zone to learn about new foods. As their confidence grows and their anxiety decreases, the more formal guidance decreases, too, and the child becomes more confident in doing hard things. A graded and compassionate push should never be used to make a child do anything. Instead, it's meant to guide the child in choosing what they are capable of, even if it feels a bit scary at first.

The Anxious Eater

We all have anxiety about trying new things. Anxious feelings are an essential alert while we consider if a new situation is safe. However, when the anxiety is out of proportion to the situation, these uncomfortable feelings get in the way of day-to-day functioning. Tantrums are part of typical development in toddlers, but frequent meltdowns are not. The difference lies in the child's ability to recover and move on with loving guidance from an adult. For example, when children have a meltdown—sobbing and screaming over green beans on their plate, unable to recover while escalating with intensity—the reaction is out of proportion to the situation. The fear is real for that child, and we don't want to dismiss that, but there is no actual danger to having a vegetable on our plate. Anxious eaters are rigid and often have strong emotions about new food encounters, even visual ones! It's not the green beans they fear, it's the prospect of having to eat them.

Cognitive behavioral therapy (CBT) is the only evidence-based therapy to address extremely anxious behaviors and anxiety disorders. Feeding specialists may collaborate with psychologists who specialize in CBT to help the most anxious children. (They may use less of the cognitive aspect of CBT for younger children but will still address anxiety even in preschoolers.) In my own work collaborating with Dr. Jonathan Dalton, founder and director of the Center for Anxiety and Behavioral Change, I've learned that when children have big emotional outbursts, it's a protective mechanism to avoid the anxious feelings more than the food itself. The problem is that anxiety *feeds* on avoidance. Every time a child avoids a food interaction in order to avoid the feelings of anxiety, that fuels their anxiety monster. By avoiding new food experiences at any level, the child is nourishing the anxiety monster and helping it thrive. As the monster gets stronger, the anxious feelings grow more intense, and the child becomes more rigid to avoid the discomfort.

For many children, eating feels like a very hard task. Building skill and ability is important, but no child will try a new food if we don't also help them learn to manage the anxiety that comes with learning to do hard things. The key to successful feeding therapy with a highly anxious child is to gently nudge them to take the next step if they have the ability but are too scared to do it on their own. It will never work to make a child do anything. The subtle difference is to support the child and help them find the courage to take that step. Therapists may incorporate deep breathing or other methods of body and brain regulation as the child learns to feel a bit of anxiety and courageously touch a new food, smell it, or perhaps lick it for the first time. Think of feeding therapy as climbing many rungs on a ladder. We take tiny steps upward, pausing frequently to breathe and take in the new sights while adjusting to unfamiliar sensations, and then we step up to the next rung. The therapist is there to guide the child, helping them feel safe and confident in their decisions to step up and out of their comfort zone.

Holly Knotowicz is an SLP and feeding specialist currently in private practice with over eleven years' experience at one of the top children's hospitals in the United States. As a young child, Holly had a PFD (pediatric feeding disorder) and a feeding tube, and encountered professionals who were extremely assertive in their techniques and unsuccessful in their efforts to help her find joy in food. Those professionals utilized more of a "shove" to get her to eat, whereas Holly and I prefer what I term "the gentle push." Both could be defined as pressure, which may seem counterintuitive when discussing responsive feeding. Kids who are in feeding therapy along with their families receive customized treatment plans to help them get to a comfortable place in the responsive feeding model. Parents and clinicians alike strive to help our children and clients develop their autonomy and internal drive to want to try new foods. Many times, children with complex medical histories require a gentle push. As a child, Holly had an underlying diagnosis that made the effort of eating extremely challenging and scary for her. She recognizes that this population of children benefits from that gentle push to overcome the fear and trauma they have experienced and associated with eating.

ADVICE FROM AN EXPERT FEEDING SPECIALIST

When working with infants and children who associate only noxious events, pain, or discomfort with feeding, the goal of fostering the internal drive to interact with new foods can be complicated. For example, children may frequently vomit due to uncontrolled gastroesophageal reflux disease (GERD), food allergies, or a diagnosis of food protein-induced enterocolitis syndrome (FPIES). When these children eat food, preferred or nonpreferred, they may associate the act of eating with vomiting. Even when the cause of the medical condition or trauma is removed or resolved, these children continue to fear any new interactions with foods. The anxiety contributes to difficulty building on feeding development and expanding the children's variety of foods, increasing the volume of food, and advancing their oral motor skills.

When identifying a "gentle push," therapists continue to follow responsive feeding strategies, sometimes integrating minor external reinforcements to rebuild and repair the child's relationship with food. For example, if a child has a history of vomiting, we continue to read the child's cues and begin to teach that child how to read their own body signals. While respecting the child from a developmental and emotional standpoint, we then provide a gentle push without providing significant pressure. There are several ways to entice interactions with foods that are also representative of that gentle push. These activities include grocery shopping with the family, helping with meal preparations, engaging in pretend play with foods, imaginary restaurant play, role playing/role switching, having fun, and being silly! For children who have significant medical trauma that is associated with the act of eating, other mild, external reinforcers may be used successfully, including games or reading books. These reinforcers can be faded out once the child's relationship with food has begun to be repaired. All these strategies are used to decrease the child's anxiety and fear, associate positive experiences with food and eating, and build confidence in food interactions.

Reading and responding to the child's cues throughout the feeding experience are important to ensure success. Treatment strategies are always individualized and in the child's best interest. Consultation with a psychologist or social worker may also be beneficial. When children learn in an environment that fosters trust and predictability, they will thrive.

Autism and Selective Eating

Mealtimes with a child who has autism can be extremely challenging. It has recently been reported that between 46 to 89 percent of children with autism have some form of food selectivity.[6] Parents worry about their child's nutritional health when their wheelhouse of foods is limited by strong preferences based on texture, color, or even the specific brand or color of the packaging it came in! Eating at restaurants or in the school cafeteria may be problematic due to the sensory overload that these kids experience in crowded environments. Social gatherings may be stigmatizing when onlookers don't understand the complexities of autism.[7] Over the past twenty years, I've learned valuable lessons from these kids and their families. My interest in helping them includes collaboration with other professionals, including board-certified behavior analysts. Nissa Goldberg, MA, BCBA, is one of the professionals I trust to provide compassionate support to help autistic children eat and thrive. Nissa shared her thoughts on the complex nature of feeding difficulties when a child has autism, explaining that these children think about the foods they eat as being in a tightly closed "box."[8]

ADVICE FROM AN EXPERT BEHAVIOR ANALYST

If a food is in the box, it is safe, well-known, and predictable. However, if a food is outside the box, it will be met with protests. Our challenge is to figure out how we can slowly crack open that box to allow new items in, little by little. Preference develops over time, so if we can just get a small amount of food to be comfortably accepted, and practice it multiple times, most kids will learn to enjoy the new food experience. The challenge is, how do we get those first couple of bites accepted?

When working with children with autism, it can be essential to use external motivation and positive reinforcement to support their encounters with novel food. The treatment plans include creating predictable routines that facilitate step-by-step progress so that over time, parents can shift to a responsive feeding model when appropriate.

Here are some gentle but effective behavioral strategies that can be implemented in a daily routine with the guidance of a professional. The following information is just to paint a picture of what behavioral therapy may look like and should not be used in place of one-on-one professional guidance.

- Pick a time to introduce novel foods outside of mealtimes. Choose a time when the child is a little hungry, but not so hungry that they will demand a preferred food.

- Choose a food that is similar, but different. We do not want to change the "safe" foods they already eat. We run the risk of "tainting" the safe food, which could lead to total rejection.

- Keep the food presentation small! Too much of a new food can be overwhelming. Start with a pea-size bite.

- When the bite is accepted, immediately provide a tangible reward (e.g., 10 seconds playing with a favorite toy) and always give verbal praise that your child enjoys. Some children are overwhelmed by big fanfare and do best with a warm smile, while others love high fives and fist bumps! The key is for you as the parent to be more fun than the reward, which will be faded out of the scenario as quickly as possible. But you will always be part of your child's feeding scenario, especially once the shift is made to a responsive feeding model after preliminary feeding treatment.

- Over the next few days, gradually increase the size and quantity of the bites while continuing to offer reinforcement. (A few tastes is the goal, and honoring a child's cues of fullness is essential.)

- The goal is that the new food, in and of itself, is a pleasant and enjoyable experience, and the external motivators are no longer needed.

Other important strategies:

- When challenging behaviors arise, do your best to ignore them. Attend only to the positive behaviors we want to see!

- It is important to rotate through both "safe" and novel foods to prevent burnout.

- Keep the mealtime structured to ensure that you are building hunger and keeping a predictable routine.

Person-first versus identity-first language

When referring to a person who has a disability, like autism, words matter. Recently, many older children and adults in the autism community have begun to request a shift from person-first (a child with autism) to identity-first language (an autistic child). The preference for one approach over the other may differ from one family to another. Some explain that we don't want to define someone by their diagnosis (person-first) while others feel that autism is an inherent part of that person's identity and something to be proud of (identity-first). To honor both preferences, I have used both options in this chapter.

Toddlers with Vision Impairment

For children who have vision impairments and feeding challenges, early intervention is critical.

Zoe Morgese, a speech therapist at the Anchor Center for Blind Children in Colorado, shared the following information:

ADVICE FROM AN EXPERT SPEECH THERAPIST

Young children with a visual impairment may be at a higher risk for experiencing challenges with feeding skills. Learning early feeding skills such as opening the mouth for a breast, bottle, or spoon are largely visual skills. Later skills such as chewing, picking up finger foods, and using utensils also depend on the many examples young children are given as they watch adults or other children at each mealtime. Children with a visual impairment, even without other structural or other medical concerns, may need intervention and designated strategies to learn and incorporate the many skills that are necessary for safe, healthy, and happy mealtimes.[9]

Based on the experience of experts like Morgese, some strategies may be helpful in facilitating the development of feeding skills in young children with visual impairment. You can try:

- using a hand-under-hand approach to introducing foods and other mealtime skills
- preparing the child verbally and/or with a touch cue for each step of the meal (e.g., "Your next bite is ready, here it comes, 1-2-3-open!")
- establishing a consistent routine in utensil placement

It's also helpful to read your young child's nonverbal cues that might communicate messages such as "done" and "I'm ready for more" and to provide sufficient wait time for the child to respond or take a turn.

It is essential to note that each child's needs must be assessed individually to determine which strategies are appropriate based on the degree and type of their visual impairment as well as on the presence of any other conditions that may affect feeding skills. These may include structural differences, sensory processing disorders, and motor delays, among others. A common strategy suggested for some children with low vision is to use a plate and/or utensil that contrasts highly in color with the foods that are being presented. Using a bright blue divided picnic plate would provide a color contrast to a meal such as mashed potatoes, shredded chicken, and mandarin orange slices. However, this suggestion would not be helpful for a child with no vision and may not be helpful in serving a meal with foods with varying colors. It also may stop being a helpful strategy if the family becomes interested in helping their child begin to use a variety of plates for social or educational reasons.

Strategies can be selected by working with a child's medical team and with a Speech/Language Pathologist or Occupational Therapist with experience with feeding skills and children with visual impairment.10 Facilitating the development of feeding skills in young children with visual impairment requires ongoing observation and, if concerns are noted, highly individualized intervention with the support of trained therapists and teachers. The future is bright for children with support and intervention.

Children with Down Syndrome

Every year, 1 in every 700 babies are born with Down syndrome.[11] It "remains the most common chromosomal condition diagnosed in the United States," according to the CDC.[12] Throughout my years as a feeding specialist, I've had the pleasure of working with children with many unique, special needs, but I have to confess that the kids with Down syndrome hold a special place in my heart! They make amazing progress, despite being challenged by obstacles like delayed motor skills, gastrointestinal issues, hearing loss, and language delays. With the support of top experts in the field, including Lori Overland, MS CCC-SLP, and Jill Rabin, MS, CCC-SLP/IBCLC, I have had the joy of watching these amazing kids thrive! Jill is the creator of Adapted Baby-Led Weaning and has years of expertise helping children with Down syndrome. Jill shared her insight on how feeding therapy requires a combination of gentle facilitation of hand-to-mouth skills using adaptive devices and other therapy strategies, while still respecting the child's communication cues.

ADVICE FROM AN EXPERT ON DOWN SYNDROME

For babies with Down syndrome, feeding may be a challenge in the first year due to low muscle tone, medical comorbidities such as heart or GI issues, and motor challenges. Experts need to start working with these babies from birth to establish a strong gross-motor base that will help create a strong foundation for optimal feeding skills. From birth, your baby's medical team should be creating a sensory-motor program to responsively work on areas such as jaw strength, lip closure, tongue elevation and lateralization, and closed-mouth resting posture. If you have a baby with Down syndrome, your therapist will create a prefeeding program to develop specific oral skills, perhaps before food is even introduced.[13] An example of a prefeeding skill that might be addressed is by having the parent place their finger where the baby's first molar would be to practice a munching pattern prior to the baby ever starting solids. A feeding therapist will also help establish a strong motor foundation and strengthen their posture in anticipation of starting solids down the road.

As babies with Down syndrome will have gross-motor delays, they may need to begin solid food feedings slightly later than their neurotypical peers. If they can attain a stable posture while well positioned in supportive seating that includes an adjustable footrest, they can begin to explore food and practice bringing hand to mouth with gentle and responsive help by the feeder (usually the parent). This is referred to as adapted baby-led weaning.[14] In the first three months, the focus is on learning about—and exploring—food, and not on food volume intake. The pressure is off! By using this adapted method, which involves using "bridge devices" such as silicone feeders, pre-loaded spoons, frozen straws, and meltable solids, as well as initial assistance of hand to mouth by the feeder/parent, those babies with Down syndrome will begin to develop improved gross-motor abilities and hand-to-mouth skill. Their improved motor skills develop due to frequent practice from the onset of starting solids. In the beginning, they will require assistance in bringing food strips, food teethers, and bridge devices to their mouth, which parents can provide with gentle guidance at the wrist. Before guiding baby's hand, wait for them to give permission by either gazing at the food, leaning toward the food, or opening their mouth for the food. This transitional period, where the caregiver helps the child bring food to their mouth, is temporary until the baby can do it themselves, eventually self-feeding just like their neurotypical peers!

Conclusion

Learning to become an adventurous eater doesn't end on a child's third birthday. In fact, the preschool years have been shown to be vital to continue to promote a child's love for all kinds of foods, especially fruits and vegetables.

I hope that you'll continue your family's journey with regular trips to the farmers market, discovering new fruits and veggies in the produce aisle, gardening and cooking together, and exploring all kinds of foods! The scope of deliciousness should include desserts and sweets, too. (I love dessert!)

Let's not think about food as good or bad. Food is food! You've raised a little person who has learned to listen to their body and respond with what it needs. Trust in all the good work that you've done and the nutritious balance you've presented while bonding with your child at mealtimes.

Continue to nurture your child's interest in joyful food interactions at family mealtimes while focusing on the most important thing: communication around the family table. When we keep our sights on nurturing communication, then responsive feeding becomes a part of our family culture for a lifetime.

Acknowledgments

My heartfelt thanks:

To the publishing team at The Experiment, who embraced my idea of writing about responsive feeding with such excitement and enthusiasm! I am grateful for the support of publisher Matthew Lore, publicist Jennifer Hergenroeder, editorial assistant Michael Ripa, and cover designer Beth Bugler. Special thanks to my fearless editor, Batya Rosenblum, who gave me expert guidance every step of the way—and always with a smile!

To Dani and her girls—the best food explorers I know!

To the many professionals who provided expert advice throughout the book, thank you for coming along on this glorious journey!

To Dr. Mitchell Katz, for being an advocate for kids with feeding difficulties and doing so with such authenticity: I am honored that you wrote the foreword for this book and am so grateful for your and Linda's friendship.

To Matthew Clyde and his mom, Melissa, who reminded me throughout 2020 that I can do hard things and do so with love.

To the families that trust me to help their children find the joy in food. What a thrill to see them become confident little food explorers, each and every one!

And finally, to my husband, Bob, and my kids, Mallory, Carly, and my son-in-law, Andrew. You know me better than anyone else and know how much I want to share my love for kids and food with the world. This book would never be possible without you saying, "You can do it," and indeed, I did. I love you.

Appendix: Resources & Recommended Products

Websites

Family Feeding and Nutrition

doctoryum.org
kidseatincolor.com
kidfoodexplorers.com
mamaknowsnutrition.com
sarahmorannutrition.com
theclinicdietitian.com
veggiesandvirtue.com

Feeding and Sensory Difficulties

feedeatspeak.co.uk
feedingmatters.com
nextstepfeeding.com
pediatricfeedingnews.com
pickyeaters.co
sensorysmarts.com

Speech and Language Concerns/Thumb and Pacifier Habits

cariebertseminars.com
geddestherapies.com
graceful-expression.com
talktools.com

Feeding Tools: Bibs, Utensils, Bowls, Plates, High Chairs, and More

ezpzfun.com
grabease.com
lollaland.com
numnumbaby.us

Shop Melanie's Amazon.com store for a variety of options for high chairs, fun tools for toddlers to use in the kitchen, child-safe knives, chewies, oral motor tools, and more: amazon.com/shop /mymunchbug.

Notes

Introduction

1. Engle, P. L., and Pelto, G. H., "Responsive feeding: implications for policy and program implementation," *The Journal of Nutrition* 141, no. 3 (2011): 508–11.

Chapter One

2. "Starting Solid Foods," HealthyChildren.org, last modified March 17, 2021, healthychildren.org/English/ages-stages/baby/feeding-nutrition/Pages/Starting-Solid-Foods.aspx.

   "Infant and young child feeding," World Health Organization, last modified June 9, 2021, who.int/news-room/fact-sheets/detail/infant-and-young-child-feeding.

3. "Vitamin D & Iron Supplements for Babies: AAP Recommendations," HealthyChildren.org, last modified May 27, 2016, healthychildren.org/English/ages-stages/baby/feeding-nutrition/Pages/Vitamin-Iron-Supplements.aspx.

4. Callahan, A., *Science of Mom: A Research-Based Guide to Your Baby's First Year* (Johns Hopkins University Press, 2021), 167.

5. Ludvigsson, J. F., and Fasano, A., "Timing of introduction of gluten and celiac disease risk," *Annals of Nutrition & Metabolism* 60, Suppl 2 (2012): 22–29.

Norris, J. M., et al., "Risk of celiac disease autoimmunity and timing of gluten introduction in the diet of infants at increased risk of disease," *JAMA* 293, no. 19 (2005): 2343–51.

Størdal, K., et al., "Early feeding and risk of celiac disease in a prospective birth cohort," *Pediatrics* 132, no. 5 (2013): e1202–9.

6. Frederiksen, B., et al., "Infant exposures and development of type 1 diabetes mellitus: The Diabetes Autoimmunity Study in the Young (DAISY)," *JAMA Pediatrics* 167, no. 9 (2013): 808–15.

Norris, J. M., et al., "Timing of initial cereal exposure in infancy and risk of islet autoimmunity," *JAMA* 290, no. 13 (2003): 1713–20.

Ziegler, A. G., et al., "Early infant feeding and risk of developing type 1 diabetes-associated autoantibodies," *JAMA* 290, no. 13 (2003): 1721–28.

7. Gaufin, T., et al., "The importance of the microbiome in pediatrics and pediatric infectious diseases," *Current Opinion in Pediatrics* 30, no. 1 (2018): 117–124.

8. Harris, G., and Mason, S. "Are There Sensitive Periods for Food Acceptance in Infancy?," *Current Nutrition Reports* 6, no. 2 (2017): 190–96.

9. Carruth, B. R., et al., "Prevalence of picky eaters among infants and toddlers and their caregivers' decisions about offering a new food," *Journal of the American Dietetic Association* 104, Suppl 1 (2004): s57–64.

10. Gisel, E. G., "Effect of food texture on the development of chewing of children between six months and two years of age," *Developmental Medicine and Child Neurology* 33, no. 1 (1991): 69–79.

11. Da Costa, S. P., et al., "Exposure to texture of foods for 8-month-old infants: Does the size of the pieces matter?," *Journal of Texture Studies* 48, no. 6 (2017): 534–40.

12. Northstone, K., et al., "The effect of age of introduction to lumpy solids on foods eaten and reported feeding difficulties at 6 and 15 months," *Journal of Human Nutrition and Dietetics: The Official Journal of the British Dietetic Association* 14, no. 1 (2001): 43–54.

13. Shaker, C., "Reading the Feeding," The ASHA Leader, last modified February 1, 2013, leader.pubs.asha.org/doi/full/10.1044/leader .FTR1.18022013.42.

14. Ibid.

15. Ibid.

16. Black, M. M., and Aboud, F. E., "Responsive feeding is embedded in a theoretical framework of responsive parenting," *The Journal of Nutrition* 141, no. 3 (2011): 490–94.

17. Ibid.

18. U.S. Department of Agriculture and U.S. Department of Health and Human Services, *Dietary Guidelines for Americans, 2020-2025*, 9th Edition, December 2020. Available at DietaryGuidelines.gov.

19. Ahishakiye, J., et al., "Challenges and responses to infant and young child feeding in rural Rwanda: A qualitative study," *Journal of Health, Population and Nutrition* 38, no. 43 (2019).

20. Ripton, N., and Potock, M., *Baby Self-Feeding: Solid food Solutions to Create Lifelong, Healthy Eating Habits* (Beverly, MA: Fair Winds, 2016), 68.

21. Potock, M., "5 Myths and Truths About Choking," Leader Live, ASHA Wire, last modified June 22, 2016, leader.pubs.asha.org/do/ 10.1044/5-myths-and-truths-about-choking/full.

22. "Choking Prevention," HealthyChildren.org, last modified September 30, 2019, healthychildren.org/English/health-issues/ injuries-emergencies/Pages/Choking-Prevention.aspx.

23. Biel, L., and Peske, N. K., *Raising a Sensory Smart Child: The Definitive Handbook for Helping Your Child with Sensory Processing Issues* (New York: Penguin Books, 2018).

24. Llewellyn, C., and Syrad, H., *An Appetite for Life: How to Feed Your Child from the Start* (New York: The Experiment, 2019), 202–5.

25. Hodges, E. A., et al., "Development of the responsiveness to child feeding cues scale," *Appetite* 65 (2013): 210–19.

26. Jenco, M., "AHA: Limit children's sugar consumption to 6 teaspoons per day," AAP News, last modified August 23, 2016, aappublications .org/news/2016/08/23/Sugar082316.

27. Hirsch, J., "Arsenic and Lead Are in Your Fruit Juice: What You Need to Know," Consumer Reports, last modified January 30, 2019, consumerreports.org/food-safety/arsenic-and-lead-are-in-your-fruit-juice-what-you-need-to-know.

28. Heyman, M. B., and Abrams, S. A., "Fruit juice in infants, children, and adolescents: Current recommendations," *Pediatrics* 139, no. 6 (2017).

29. "Listeriosis Infection," HealthyChildren.org, last modified November 21, 2015, healthychildren.org/English/health-issues/conditions/infections/Pages/Listeriosis-Infection.aspx.

30. LaMotte, S., "Leading baby food manufacturers knowingly sold products with high levels of toxic metals, a congressional investigation found," CNN Health, February 5, 2021.

31. "Heavy Metals in Baby Food," HealthyChildren.org, last modified September 6, 2021, healthychildren.org/English/ages-stages/baby/feeding-nutrition/Pages/Metals-in-Baby-Food.aspx.

32. Ibid.

33. Ibid.

34. "Common Allergens," FARE, foodallergy.org/living-food-allergies/food-allergy-essentials/common-allergens. Accessed December 28, 2020.

35. "Safe Minimum Internal Temperature Chart," U.S. Department of Agriculture, Food Safety and Inspection Service, fsis.usda.gov/food-safety/safe-food-handling-and-preparation/food-safety-basics/safe-temperature-chart. Accessed December 28, 2020.

36. Ibid.

37. Fernando, N., and Potock, M., *Raising a Healthy, Happy Eater: A Parent's Handbook—A Stage-by-Stage Guide to Setting Your Child on the Path to Adventurous Eating* (New York: The Experiment, 2015), 44.

38. Clayton, H. B., et al., "Prevalence and reasons for introducing infants early to solid foods: Variations by milk feeding type," *Pediatrics* 131, no. 4 (2013): e1108–14.

Chapter Two

1. Piazza, E. A., et al., "Mothers consistently alter their unique vocal fingerprints when communicating with infants," *Current Biology* 27 (2017): 3162–67.

2. "What Is Speech? What Is Language?," American Speech-Language-Hearing Association, asha.org/public/speech/development/ speech-and-language. Accessed February 6, 2021.

3. "Birth to One Year," American Speech-Language-Hearing Association, asha.org/public/speech/development/01. Accessed February 6, 2021.

4. Ibid.

5. "Infant and young child feeding," World Health Organization, last modified June 9, 2021, who.int/news-room/fact-sheets/detail/ infant-and-young-child-feeding.

6. Zimmels, S., email to the author.

7. Hayes, D., "Feeding Vegetarian and Vegan Infants and Toddlers," Eat Right, Academy of Nutrition and Dietetics, last modified October 23, 2019, eatright.org/food/nutrition/vegetarian-and-special-diets/ feeding-vegetarian-and-vegan-infants-and-toddlers.

8. Potock, M., *Adventures in Veggieland: Help Your Kids Learn to Love Vegetables with 100 Easy Activities and Recipes* (New York: The Experiment LLC, 2018), 9.

9. Fernando and Potock, *Raising a Healthy, Happy Eater*, op. cit.

10. Potock, M., "Step Away from the Sippy Cup!," Leader Live, ASHA Wire, last modified January 8. 2014, leader.pubs.asha.org/do/10.1044/ step-away-from-the-sippy-cup/full.

11. Fernando and Potock, *Raising a Healthy, Happy Eater*, op. cit.

12. Sexton, S., and Natale, R., "Risks and benefits of pacifiers," *American Family Physician* 79, no. 8 (2009): 681–85.

Chapter Three

1. "Is Your Baby Hungry or Full? Responsive Feeding Explained," HealthyChildren.org, last modified September 1, 2017, healthychildren .org/English/ages-stages/baby/feeding-nutrition/Pages/Is-You r-Baby-Hungry-or-Full-Responsive-Feeding-Explained.aspx.

2. Gasparro, A., "Falling Sales Squeeze Baby-Food Pouches," *The Wall Street Journal*, December 23, 2019.

3. Cernansky, R., "Rethinking Baby Food Pouches," *The New York Times*, June 19, 2018.

4. Potock, M., "The Great Pouch Debate: Pros, Cons and Compromising," Leader Live, ASHA Wire, last modified March 29, 2017, leader .pubs.asha.org/do/10.1044/the-great-pouch-debate-pros- cons-and-compromising/full.

5. Cording, J., "Do Kids Need Omega 3 Fats?," Eat Right, Academy of Nutrition and Dietetics, last modified August 12, 2020, eatright.org/ food/vitamins-and-supplements/types-of-vitamins-and-nutrients/ do-kids-need-omega-3-fats.

6. "What About Fat and Cholesterol?," HealthyChildren.org, last modified July 25, 2018, healthychildren.org/English/healthy-living/nutrition/ Pages/What-About-Fat-And-Cholesterol.aspx.

7. "How Much Fiber Do Children Need?," Cleveland Clinic, last modified December 30, 2020, health.clevelandclinic.org/ figuring-dietary-fiber-child-need.

8. "How Much Water Should Kids Drink?," CHOC, choc.org/ programs-services/urology/how-much-water-should-my-child-drink. Accessed March 9, 2021.

9. Muth, N. D., "Recommended Drinks for Young Children Ages 0–5," HealthyChildren.org, last modified September 18, 2019, healthychildren.org/English/healthy-living/nutrition/Pages/ Recommended-Drinks-for-Young-Children-Ages-0-5.aspx.

10. Ibid.

11. Fadda, R., et al., "Effects of drinking supplementary water at school on cognitive performance in children," *Appetite* 59, no. 3 (2012): 730–37.

12. Muth, HealthyChildren.org, op. cit.

13. "Where We Stand: Fruit Juice," HealthyChildren.org, last modified May 19, 2017, healthychildren.org/English/healthy-living/nutrition/Pages/Where-We-Stand-Fruit-Juice.aspx.

14. Thacher, T. D., et al., "Increasing incidence of nutritional rickets: a population-based study in Olmsted County, Minnesota," *Mayo Clinic Proceedings* 88, no. 2 (2013): 176–183.

15. "Advice about Eating Fish," U.S. Food & Drug Administration, www.fda.gov/food/consumers/advice-about-eating-fish. Accessed March 10, 2021.

16. Al-Shawwa, B., et al., "Vitamin D and sleep in children," *Journal of Clinical Sleep Medicine* 16, no. 7 (2020): 1119–23.

17. Fernando, N., email to the author, March 10, 2021.

18. "Constipation," GI Kids, gikids.org/constipation/?fbclid=IwAR34ilK7BpakGP3aYX1gt6r1LZV5vzXGqTBV55LSB5UocxPaRU1lXq2En6I. Accessed March 10, 2021.

19. Chao, H. C., et al., "The Impact of Constipation on Growth in Children," *Pediatric Research* 64 (2008): 308–11.

20. Ramos-Jorge, J., et al., "Prospective longitudinal study of signs and symptoms associated with primary tooth eruption," *Pediatrics* 128, no. 3 (2011): 471–76.

   Macknin, M.L., et al., "Symptoms associated with infant teething: a prospective study," *Pediatrics* 105, no. 4, pt. 1 (2000): 747–52.

21. "Safely Soothing Teething Pain and Sensory Needs in Babies and Older Children," U.S. Food & Drug Administration, www.fda.gov/consumers/consumer-updates/safely-soothing-teething-pain-and-sensory-needs-babies-and-older-children. Accessed April 12, 2021.

22. "Teething: Tips for soothing sore gums," Mayo Clinic, last modified January 9, 2020, mayoclinic.org/healthy-lifestyle/infant-and-toddler-health/in-depth/teething/art-20046378.

23. Hunter Lopez, L., "The trouble With Amber Teething Necklaces," *The New York Times*, last modified April 18, 2020, nytimes.com/2020/04/18/parenting/amber-teething-necklaces.html.

24. Fernando and Potock, *Raising a Healthy, Happy Eater*, op. cit.

25. Geddes, E., email to the author, March 3, 2021.

Chapter Four

1. Bernales, G., email to the author, March 6, 2021.

2. Ibid.

3. Ibid.

4. Ibid.

5. Fernando and Potock, *Raising a Healthy, Happy Eater*, op. cit.

6. "Developmental Milestones 18 to 24 Months," Children's Minnesota, last modified June 2015, childrensmn.org/educationmaterials/ childrensmn/article/15315/developmental-milestones-18-to-24-months.

7. McCloy, M., email to the author, March 24, 2021.

8. Creskoff Maune, N., email to the author, April 11, 2021.

9. "Late Language Emergence," American Speech-Language-Hearing Association, asha.org/practice-portal/clinical-topics/ late-language-emergence. Accessed April 13, 2021.

Chapter Five

1. Shafer, L., "Summertime, Playtime," Usable Knowledge, Harvard Graduate School of Education, last modified June 12, 2018, gse.harvard .edu/news/uk/18/06/summertime-playtime.

2. Lowry, L., "The Land of Make Believe: How and Why to Encourage Pretend Play," The Hanen Centre, hanen.org/helpful-info/articles/ the-land-of-make-believe.aspx. Accessed April 9, 2021.

3. Lumeng, J. C., et al., "Picky eating, pressuring feeding, and growth in toddlers," *Appetite* 123 (2018): 299–305.

4. Baker-Smith, C. M., et al., "The use of nonnutritive sweeteners in children," *Pediatrics* 144, no. 5 (2019).

5. "Study finds inadequate hydration among U.S. children," Harvard T. H. Chan School of Public Health, last modified June 11, 2015, hsph .harvard.edu/news/press-releases/study-finds-inadequate-hydration-among-u-s-children.

6. Kenney, E. L., et al., "Prevalence of Inadequate Hydration among US Children and Disparities by Gender and Race/Ethnicity: National Health and Nutrition Examination Survey, 2009–2012," *American Journal of Public Health* 105, no. 8 (2015): e113–18.

7. Potock, M., "5 Fun Ways to Get Kids Drinking More Water," Leader Live, ASHA Wire, last modified October 12, 2016, leader.pubs.asha.org/do/10.1044/5-fun-ways-to-get-kids-drinking-more-water/full.

8. Hammons, A. J., and Fiese, B. H., "Is frequency of shared family meals related to the nutritional health of children and adolescents?," *Pediatrics* 127, no. 6 (2011): e1565–74.

9. Snow, C. E., and Beals, D. E., "Mealtime talk that supports literacy development," *New Directions for Child and Adolescent Development* 2006, no. 111 (2006): 51–66.

10. Potock, *Adventures in Veggieland*, op. cit.

11. Fishel, A., "The most important thing you can do with your kids? Eat dinner with them," *The Washington Post*, January 12, 2015.

12. Snow and Beals, *New Directions for Child and Adolescent Development*, op. cit.

    "Research shows family dinner improves literacy," The Family Dinner Project, last modified August 31, 2020, thefamilydinnerproject.org/blog/research-shows-family-dinner-improves-literacy.

13. Suggate, S., et al., "From infancy to adolescence: The longitudinal links between vocabulary, early literacy skills, oral narrative, and reading comprehension," *Cognitive Development* 47 (2018): 82–95.

14. Hofferth, S. L., and Sandberg, J. F., "How American children spend their time," *Journal of Marriage and Family* 63, no. 2 (2001): 295–308.

15. Fishel, A., "Science says: eat with your kids," The Conversation, last modified January 9, 2015, theconversation.com/science-says-eat-with-your-kids-34573.

Chapter Six

1. Lebovitz, D., email to the author, March 14, 2021.

2. Koerner, A. F., et al., "Understanding Family Communication Patterns and Family Functioning: The Roles of Conversation Orientation and Conformity Orientation," *Annals of the International Communication Association* 26, no. 1 (2002): 37–69.

3. Hazan, S., email to the author, March 4, 2021.

4. Cannon, W., email to the author, March 21, 2021.

Chapter Seven

1. Tai-Seale, M., et al., "Time allocation in primary care office visits," *Health Services Research* 42, no. 5 (2007): 1871–94.

2. Benjasuwantep, B., et al., "Feeding problems in healthy young children: prevalence, related factors and feeding practices," *Pediatric Reports* 5, no. 2 (2013): 38–42.

3. "The Seven Cs of Communication," Education Executive, last modified June 28, 2017, edexec.co.uk/the-seven-cs-of-communication.

4. Chatoor, I., et al., "Feeding development and disorders," *Encyclopedia of Infant and Early Childhood Development* (New York: Academic Press, 2008), 524–33.

5. Aviram, I., et al., "Mealtime Dynamics in Child Feeding Disorder: The Role of Child Temperament, Parental Sense of Competence, and Paternal Involvement," *Journal of Pediatric Psychology* 40, no., 1 (2014): 45–54.

6. Ledford, J. R., and Gast, D. L., "Feeding Problems in Children With Autism Spectrum Disorders: A Review," *Focus on Autism and Other Developmental Disabilities* 21, no. 3 (2006): 153–66.

7. Goldberg, N., email to the author, April 2, 2021.

8. Ibid.

9. Smyth, C., et al., "Family voices at mealtime: Experiences with young children with visual impairment," *Topics in Early Childhood Special Education* 34 (2014): 175–85.

10. "Mealtime Routines Visual Impairment Intervention," University of Northern Colorado, last modified September 17, 2019, go.unco.edu/mrvi.

11. Mai, C. T., et al., "National population-based estimates for major birth defects, 2010–2014," *Birth Defects Research* 111, no. 18 (2019): 1420–35.

12. "Facts about Down Syndrome," Centers for Disease Control and Prevention, last modified April 6, 2021, cdc.gov/ncbddd/birthdefects/downsyndrome.html.

13. Overland, L., and Merkel-Walsh, R., *A Sensory Motor Approach to Feeding* (TalkTools, 2013).

14. "Adapted Baby-Led Weaning for Babies with Feeding Challenges," Chicago Feeding Group, chicagofeedinggroup.thinkific.com/courses/adapted-baby-led-weaning.

Image Credits

Index

Page numbers in *italics* refer to photos.

6 months, 7–64
  concerns, common, 60–61
  feeding methods, 13–14, 15
  food to avoid, 53–55
  gagging versus choking, 29–36
  handheld solids and mashes, 22–24, *23*
  hunger versus appetite, 44–47
  myths about feeding, 62–64
  purees, debate over, 13, 18–19
  purees, offering, 19–22
  reflexes, 12, 24–29
  senses, 37–44
  solid foods, getting in groove with, 48–59
  solid foods, starting, 7–12
6 to 12 months, 65–101
  bottle weaning, 95
  challenges, common, 96–101
  choking concerns, 73–74
  communication, 65–69, 97
  cutting food for baby, *74*, 74–76
  eating times and growing times, 69–70

food groups, 76–78, *79*
food to avoid, 53–55
gums, breaking food down with, 72–73
main dishes, 80
one family, one meal concept, 72–82
pacifiers, 87, 88, 93–95
side dishes, 81
softening foods quickly, 78
solid foods, transitioning to, 70–71
tools, 82–93
12 to 18 months, 103–40
  appetite, transitions in, 119–28, *126*
  eater types, 130–33
  fingers and fists, reliance on, 105
  foods to offer, 106–7
  meal sizes, 110
  nutrition, shifts in, 112–19
  portion sizes, 109
  purees in pouches, overreliance on, 107–9
  reflexes, 103–5

12 to 18 months (*continued*)
snack sizes, 110–11
tongue, brushing, 124, 139
toothbrushing, 139
transitions, tricky, 134–40
veggie needs, 112
18 to 24 months, 141–59
language development,
141–44
mealtime transitions, 150–52
myths, feeding and
communication, 157–59
napkins, 153–54
open-cup drinking, 145–48,
147
self-feeding skills, 145–57
swallowing, 154–56
symbolic play, 144
time it takes to eat, 152–53
travel cups, 156–57
utensils, transitioning to
bigger, 148–50
vocabulary, 141–42
24 to 36 months, 161–77
cries for food, responding to,
165–66
emotions, responding,
163–64
mealtimes, family, 175–77
new foods, fear of, 167–70
"no," responding to toddler's,
161–63
responsive play, 164–65
sugar and artificial
sweeteners, 170–72
water, encouraging toddlers
to drink, 172–74

A

AAP. *See* American Academy of
Pediatrics
ABCs, responding to emotions
with, 163–64
Aboud, Frances, 16–17
Academy of Nutrition and
Dietetics, 77–78
actions, labeling, 143
adjusted age, of premature
babies, 59
Adventures in Veggieland
(Potock), 82
airplane game, 19, 20
allergenic foods, introducing,
57–59
allergic reactions, 59
American Academy of Family
Physicians, 93, 94
American Academy of
Pediatrics (AAP)
breast milk, 7–8
choking hazards, 35
formula, 116–17
grains, 56
heavy metals, avoiding, 56
pacifiers, 93
satiety cues, 47
soy milk, 116
sugar, 55
American Speech-Language-
Hearing Association (ASHA),
66–67, 158
anemia, 119
anxious eaters, 201–2
appetite
constipation and, 121–22
exercise and, 124–25
growth and, 119–21
hunger versus, 44–47
teething and, 122–23
utensils and, 125–28, 126
Appetite for Life, An (Llewellyn
& Syrad), 45–46
aquariums, homemade, 173
articulation, 26
artificial sweeteners, 171–72
ASHA (American
Speech-Language-Hearing
Association), 66–67, 158

aspiration, 34, 36, 89, 190
attention, giving/withholding, 129, 132
auditory distractions, 41
autism and selective eating, 204–6
Avent Soothie pacifiers, 93
avocado, 81
avoidance, 202

B

baby food, making own, 56
Baby-Led Weaning (BLW), 13–14, 18, 73, 100
background noise, 41
balance and movement, sense of, 43
Barnes, Kacie, 112–19
bears, tiny, 173
beginning of meals, 124–25, 150–51
behavior, 96, 199, 205–6
behavior analysts, 205–6
Beil, Lindsey, 37
bento boxes, 187
benzocaine, 123
Bernales, Grace, 142
beverages, sugary, 117
bibs, 50–51
"big scoop, small sample" strategy, 168
biting reflex, 28–29, 104
"bit of everything on our plate" concept, 168–69
Black, Maureen M., 16–17
blanching food, 78
BLISS study, 73
BLW (Baby-Led Weaning), 13–14, 18, 73, 100
BMs (bowel movements), 115, 121–22
body parts, awareness of, 43–44
bottle weaning, 95, 134–35

botulism, infant, 53
boundaries, maintaining, 163, 164
bowel movements (BMs), 115, 121–22
bracing while drinking, 156–57
bread, 36, 77
breaking pacifiers, with love, 136
breastfeeding, 134
breast milk, 7–8, 48, 53, 56
Browne, Joy V., 15
brushing inside mouth, 100

C

caffeine, 117
calcium, 117–18
Callahan, Alice, 8–9
calling 911, 33, 59
candy, hard/sticky, 35
Cannon, Wendy, 184–87
carbohydrates, 112–13
carrots, 81
Castle, Jill, 119
CBT (cognitive behavioral therapy), 201–2
Centers for Disease Control and Prevention (CDC), 195, 209
cereal, rice, 22, 56
cheese, 35, 54–55
cherry tomatoes, 75
chewing gum, 35
chewing myth, 63
chia seeds, 53
child feeding questionnaire, 198
Children's Hospital of Orange County, 115–16
chili, 80
chipmunks (eater type), 133
choices, offering, 68, 162–63, 164
choke-shields on spoons/forks, 83

choking
gagging and, 34
hazards, 35–36
myths, 32–33, 63
preventing, 30–31
responding to, 31–34, 73–74
truths, 33–34
cleanup songs, 124
clearing the table, 151–52
cognitive behavioral therapy
(CBT), 201–2
Columbia University, 176
communication
6 to 12 months, 65–69
18 to 24 months, 157–59
biting reflex and, 29
gagging reflex and, 29
myths, 157–59
with pediatricians, 196–98
rooting reflex and, 25
sign language for babies,
68–69, 97
suckling reflex and, 26
swallowing reflex and, 28
tongue reflex and, 26–27
transverse tongue reflex and,
27
community support, creating,
184
complex carbohydrates, 112–13
constipation, 115, 121–22
cooking, "sabotaging" during,
142
corn kernels, 36, 112
coughing while eating, 32, 33,
190–91
covert restriction, 45
CPR courses, infant, 31
Creskoff, Nancy, 151–52
cries for food, responding to,
165–66
cruisers (eater type), 131
cubes (food cut), 74, 75–76
cue-based feeding, 15

cultural influences, 182–84
cup fairy houses, 173–74
cups
open, 92, 145–48, 147
sippy, 86–88, 158
straw, 92–93, 135, 156–57
360, 88–90, 89
travel, 156–57
cutting food for baby, 74, 74–76,
157–58
cutting skills, 149–50

D

dairy/dairy substitutes, 58,
77–78, 79
Dalton, Jonathan, 202
day care, 184–88
deli meats, 54–55
dessert, 171, 172
developmentally supportive
care, 15
diapers, soiled, 98
diarrhea, 115
Dietary Guidelines (US
Department of Health), 18
dip, scoop, and flip motion,
126–27
dip, scoop, and turn motion, 83,
127
dip and flip motion, 83, 125–26,
127
dips, 101
disliked food, 97
distractions and wiggling, 98
Doctor Yum Preschool Food
Adventure, 184
documenting child's eating, 197
Down syndrome, 209–10
drinking
bracing while, 156–57
open-cup, 145–48, 147
straw, 87, 90–91, 135
drooling, 158

E

early intervention, 195
eater types
  anxious, 201–2
  chipmunks, 133
  cruisers, 131
  food explorers, 130–31, 187
  food throwers, 96–97
  learning, 130
  mess makers, 131–32
  overly enthusiastic, 99, 133
  picky, 167, 189, 191
  plate tossers, 97
  poopers, 132–33
  stuffers, 100–101
  wigglers, 98
"eat this, then that," 169
Ebert, Cari, 68–69
eggs, 54–55, 57, 58
emotional outbursts, 163–64, 201
end of meals, 151–52
esophageal phase of
  swallowing, 28
exercise and appetite, 124–25
expressive language, 66, 67

F

face washing, 19–20, 153–54
Family Dinner Project, The, 177
family feeding/nutrition
  websites, 213
family history, understanding,
  181
family influences, 180–84
family mealtimes, 175–77
family-style strategies, 168–69,
  170
fats, 113–14
FDA (Food and Drug
  Administration), 118, 123
fear of new foods, 167–70
feeding
  approach, discussing, 181–82
  biting reflex and, 28

cue-based, 15
gagging reflex and, 29
hybrid approach to, 14, 100
mindful, 17–18
myths, 62–64, 157–59, 189–91
physiology and, 199
rooting reflex and, 25
suckling reflex and, 25
swallowing reflex and, 28
tongue reflex and, 26
traditional, 13, 18
transverse tongue reflex and,
  27
volume-driven, 15
websites, 213–14
See also responsive feeding;
  specific topics
feeding chairs, 49–50, 50, 82,
  98, 214
feeding disorders
  about, 192–93
  anxious eaters, 201–2
  autism and, 204–6
  building blocks of, 199
  Down syndrome and, 209–10
  early intervention, 195
  feeding therapists and,
    200–204
  gentle pushes and, 200–201,
    203–4
  mealtime dynamics and,
    199–200
  pediatrician and, 194–98
  red flags, 195–96
  vision impairment and, 207–8
feeding evaluation, 115, 191, 197
feedingmatters.org, 198
feeding questionnaire, 198
feeding specialists, 182–84,
  203–4
feeding therapists, 200–204
feeding tools, 82–93, 214
feelings, acknowledging, 163,
  164

Fernando, Nimali, 121, 136, 184
fiber, 115
fibrous foods, 36
fine-motor skills, 11, 189–90, 199
fingers, using, 20–21, 105
finger sucking, 137–39, 158
first foods, 52
Fischel, Anne, 177
fish, 56, 58
fists, reliance on, 105
flavors, exposure to new, 9
flexibility, 18–19
food
  allergenic, 57–59
  baby, homemade, 56
  blanching, 78
  cries for, 165–66
  cutting, 74, 74–76, 149–50,
    157–58
  disliked, 97
  fear of new, 167–70
  fibrous, 36
  first, 52
  "grab and gab," 187
  gums, breaking down with,
    72–73
  new, fear of, 167–70
  organic, 56
  slippery, 53
  smashed, 74, 75
  softening, 78
  spitting out, 63–64
  steaming, 78
Food and Drug Administration
  (FDA), 118, 123
food explorers (eater type),
  130–31, 187
food groups, preparing, 76–78,
  79
food intolerances, 59
food throwers (eater type),
  96–97
forks, 83, 125–26, 128, 148–49
formula, 8, 48, 53, 116–17

frittatas, 80
fruits, 76, 79
frustration, 97
fussing child, 68–69

G

gagging
  about, 29–30
  choking and, 34
  concern about, 61
  myths, 32–33
  responding to, 31–34
  truths, 33–34
gagging reflex, 29
gastrocolic reflex, 98, 132
Geddes, Erin, 137–39
gentle pushes, 200–201, 203–4
Goldberg, Nissa, 205–6
"grab and gab food," 187
grains, 56, 77, 79
grapes, 35, 75
grazing, 111
greens, raw leafy, 36
gross-motor skills, 10, 11, 12, 199,
  210
growth and appetite, 119–21
growth charts, 120–21
growth curves, 121, 191
gum, chewing, 35
gums, breaking food down
  with, 72–73
gustatory sense, 41, 42–43

H

habits, modeling good, 174
handheld solids, 22–24, 23
hand preference, 128
Hanen Center, 165
Harvard Graduate School of
  Education, 164
Harvard T. H. Chan School of
  Public Health, 172
Hazan, Sophia, 182–84
health and family meals, 175

hearing, 40–41
heavy metals, 55–57
heritage, flavors of your, 182–84
high chairs, 49–50, *50*, 82, 98, 214
homeopathic teething tablets,
    123
honey, 45, 53
honey bears, 173
hot dogs, 35
hot items, teacher opening of,
    187
hunger cues, 46–47, 48
hunger versus appetite, 44–47
hybrid approach to feeding, 14,
    100

I

ice pops, homemade, 123
identity-first language, 207
imitation, 66, 67
immune system, 8–9
infant botulism, 53
infant CPR courses, 31
infant-directed speech, 65–66
insoluble fiber, 115
intelligence and family meals,
    175–76
internal cues, sense of, 44
internal distractions, 98
interoception, 44
iron, 118–19
iron supplements, 8

J

Jacobson, Maryanne, 119
jewelry for teething pain, 123
Jewish culture, 183
Journal of Pediatric Psychology,
    199
juice, 54, 117, 118

K

Katz, Mitchell, 189
kidneys, 54

kids' menus, restaurant, 188
knives, 149–50
Knotowicz, Holly, 203–4

L

language
    expressive, 66, 67
    mealtimes and, 142–44,
        175–76
    person-first versus
        identity-first, 207
    receptive, 66, 67, 143–44
    sense of sight and, 38–39
    sense of smell and, 41–42
    sense of sound and, 40
    sense of taste and, 42–43
    sense of touch and, 39–40
    speech versus, 66
    websites, 214
lasagna, 80
lead hazards in home, 57
learned behaviors, 199
learning eaters, 130
Lebovitz, Dani, 180–82
listeriosis, 54–55
Llewellyn, Clare, 45–46
loveys, 134–35, 135–36
lunches, packed, 186–88

M

Magic 1, 2, 3, 4 Method, 145–48,
    147
main dishes, 80
mashes, 22–24, *23*
master server strategy, 168
matchsticks (food cut), *74*, 75
Mayo Clinic, 123
McCloy, Mia, 149
meals
    beginning of, 124–25, 150–51
    end of, 151–52
    mini, 70
    sizes, 110

mealtimes
  asking child questions
    during, 144
  experience, describing, 69
  family, 175–77
  feeding disorders and,
    199–200
  language development
    during, 142–44, 175–76
  meditation at, 17–18
  rules for, 174
  "sabotaging" during, 142
  setting stage for happy,
    48–50
  transitions, 124–25, 150–52
meats, 35, 54–55, 76–77
"meditation at mealtimes,"
  17–18
mess makers (eater type), 131–32
messy mouth, cleaning during
  feeding, 19–20
metals, heavy, 55–57
milk
  as beverage, 53–54, 77–78,
    116
  breast, 7–8, 48, 53, 56
  plant-based, 116
mindful feeding, 17–18
mini meals, 70
modeling good habits, 174
monounsaturated fats, 114
Morgese, Zoe, 207
motherese, 65–66
motor skills
  fine, 11, 189–90, 199
  gross, 10, 11, 12
movement, sense of, 43
Murkett, Tracey, 13
myths
  communication, 157–59
  feeding, 62–64, 157–59,
    189–91
  gagging versus choking,
    32–33

purees, offering, 22
solids, starting, 12

N

napkins, 153–54
Nationwide Children's Hospital
  (Ohio), 88
neophobia, as term, 167
new foods, fear of, 167–70
nibble trays, 165–66
911, calling, 33, 59
"no," responding to toddler's,
  161–63
noise, background, 41
nonnutritive sweeteners
  (NNS), 171
North American Society for
  Pediatric Gastroenterology,
  Hepatology, and Nutrition, 121
nouns, labeling, 143
nuts, 35, 58

O

objects, labeling, 143
occupational therapists, 149,
  190, 208
olfactory sense, 41–42
omega-3, 114
omega-6, 114
omelets, 80
one family, one meal concept,
  72–82
  choking concerns, 73–74
  cutting food for baby, 74,
    74–76
  food groups, 76–78
  gums, breaking food down
    with, 72–73
  main dishes, 80
  quick prep, 79
  side dishes, 81
  softening foods quickly, 78
  at the table, 82
open cups, 92, 145–48, 147

oral myologists, 137–39
oral phase of swallowing, 28
organic foods, 56
Overland, Lori, 209
overly enthusiastic eaters, 99,
133
overstuffing, 100–101
overt restriction, 45–46

P

pacifier fairy, 136
pacifiers
6 to 12 months, 87, 88,
93–95
12 to 18 months, 135–37
18 to 24 months, 158, 159
weaning from, 94–95,
135–37
websites, 214
paci-houses, 94
packed lunches, 186–88
parenting, responsive, 16–17
peanut butter, 35, 57, 58
peanuts, 58
peas, 36, 186–87
pediatric feeding evaluation,
115, 191, 197
pediatricians, 60, 61, 190,
194–98
person-first language, 207
pharnygeal phase of
swallowing, 28
photos, to document child's
eating, 197
physiology and feeding, 199
Piaget, Jean, 144
picky eaters, 167, 189, 191
pincer grasp, 64, 85–86, 105
pinky-strips (food cut), 74, 75
pizza, 80
plates, 157, 208, 214
plate tossers (eater type), 97
play, 144, 164–65
polyunsaturated fats, 114

poopers (eater type), 132–33
popcorn, 35
portion sizes, 46, 47, 97, 109,
169
potatoes, 81
Potock, Melanie
Adventures in Veggieland,
82
*Raising a Healthy, Happy
Eater* (Fernando & Potock),
136
"Step Away from the Sippy
Cup," 86
prefeeding skills, 209
premature babies, 59
pre-plating strategies, 169–70
preschool, 184–88
pre-spoons, 51, 82–83
pretend play, 165
Princeton's Baby Lab, 65–66
proprioception, 43–44
protein, 79, 113
purees
6 months, 13, 18–19
12 to 18 months, 104, 107–9
bite reflex and, 104
debate over, 13, 18–19
making, 109
myths, 63
offering, 19–22, 84
overstuffing and, 100
in pouches, overreliance on,
107–9
spoon-feeding tips, 84–85
straw drinking, 90–91
pushes, gentle, 200–201,
203–4

Q

questionnaire, child feeding,
198
questions, asking child, 144
quiches, 80

R

Rabin, Jill, 209–10
Raising a Healthy, Happy Eater
  (Fernando & Potock), 136
Rapley, Gill, 13
RDNs (Registered Dietitian
  Nutritionists), 112–19, 170–72,
  180–82
readiness, signs of, 11–12, 60
"Reading the Feeding" (Shaker),
  15
receptive language, 66, 67,
  143–44
Red Cross, 31
red flags, 195–96
reflexes
  6 months, 12, 24–29
  12 to 18 months, 103–5
  about, 24
  biting, 28–29, 104
  gagging, 29
  gastrocolic, 98, 132
  rooting, 25
  suckling, 25–26
  swallowing, 28, 104
  tongue-protrusion, 12, 26–27,
    72–73, 84–85, 104–5
  transverse tongue, 27, 105
Registered Dietitian
  Nutritionists (RDNs), 112–19,
  170–72, 180–82
resources, 213–14
responsive feeding
  advantages of, 3–4
  author's introduction to,
    14–16
  as baby-led and
    parent-responsive, 17–18
  components, 45–46
  flexibility of, 18–19
  responsive parenting,
    similarities with, 16–17
  thriving and, 18
  See also specific topics

responsive parenting, 16–17
responsive play, 164–65
restriction, 45–46, 55
rice, 56
rice cereal, 22, 56
rickets, 118
rooting reflex, 25
Ross, Erin Sundseth, 15
rotary chew, 63, 145
rules for mealtimes, 174
runny stools, 115

S

"sabotaging," 142
safety and family meals, 176
salt, added, 54
satiety cues, 47, 97, 132
saturated fats, 114
"Say ____", 143
seeds, 35
selective eating, 204–6
self-feeding skills
  12 to 18 months, *126*, 126–27
  18 to 24 months, 145–57
  mealtime transitions, 150–52
  napkins, 153–54
  open-cup drinking, 145–48,
    147
  spoons, *126*, 126–27
  swallowing, 154–56
  time it takes to eat, 152–53
  travel cups, 156–57
  utensils, transitioning to
    bigger, 148–50
self-soothing, 159
senses, 37–44
  interoception, 44
  proprioception, 43–44
  sight, 37–39
  smell, 41–42
  sound, 40–41
  taste, 42–43
  touch, 39–40
  vestibular, 43

sensory difficulties, 207–8, 213–14
sensory distractions, 98
Sephardic Jews, 183
sesame, 58
Shaker, Catherine, 15, 19
shellfish, 58
side dishes, 81
sight, sense of, 37–39
sign language for babies, 68–69, 97
silent aspiration, 34
silicone feeders, 123
simple carbohydrates, 113
sippy cups, spouted, 86–88, 158
sleep, 62, 138
slippery foods, 53
SLPs. See speech-language pathologists
"smash cakes," 55
smashed food, 74, 75
smell, sense of, 41–42
smiling, 48, 49
Smith, Ashley, 170–71
smoking, 57
snacks, 70, 110–11
soda, 117
softening foods, 78
solid foods, starting, 7–12
soluble fiber, 115
songs, cleanup, 124
sound, sense of, 40–41
soy, 58
soy milk, 116
speech, 65–66, 214
speech-language pathologists (SLPs)
  coughing, 190–91
  gentle push, 203–4
  role of, 14
  "sabotaging," 142
  "Say ____", 143
  sign language, 68–69
  sippy cups, 87

360 cups, 88
vision impairment, 208
Spence, Charles, 41
spitting out food, 63–64
spoon-feeding tips, 83–85
spoons
  appetite and, 125, 126, 126–27
  choke-shields on, 83
  first, 51
  right-size, 83, 85
  transitioning to bigger, 148–49
sports drinks, 117
steaks, 76, 77
steaming food, 78
"Step Away from the Sippy Cup" (Potock), 86
stools, runny, 115
storytelling, 176
straw cups, 92–93, 135, 156–57
straw drinking, 87, 90–91, 135
stress reduction, 176–77
stuffers (eater type), 100–101
suckling reflex, 25–26
sugar, 54, 55, 170–71
sugar alcohols, 171
sugar snap peas, 186–87
swallowing, 63, 154–56
swallowing reflex, 28, 104
sweeteners, artificial, 171–72
sweet potatoes, 81
symbolic play, 144
Syrad, Hayley, 45–46
Syrian Jews, 183

T

table, clearing, 151–52
tactile sensations, 39–40
talkers, late, 158
tantrums, 163–64, 201
taste, sense of, 41, 42–43
teeth, 62
teethers, 136–37
teething and appetite, 122–23

teething rings, 123
teething toys, 122
tethered oral tissues, 64, 137
textures, exposure to new, 10,
    11–12
360 cups, 88–90, *89*
Three Ts method (Toothpaste,
    Target, Two!), 139
thriving, 18
thumb sucking, 137–39, 159, 214
time it takes to eat, 152–53
tomatoes, cherry, 75
tongue, brushing, 124, 139
tongue-protrusion reflex, 12,
    26–27, 72–73, 84–85, 104–5
tools, feeding, 82–93, 214
toothbrushing, 139
toothpaste, spitting out, 139
touch, sense of, 39–40
traditional feeding, 13, 18
trans fats, 114
transverse tongue reflex, 27,
    105
travel cups, 156–57
tree nuts, 58

U
US Department of Health, 18
utensils
    appetite and, 125–28
    forks, 83, 125–26, 128, 148–49
    knives, 149–50
    need for, 189–90
    pre-spoons, 51, 82–83
    transitioning to bigger,
        148–50
    See also spoons

V
vaping, 57
vegetables
    6 months, 35, 52
    6 to 12 months, 76, 79
    12 to 18 months, 112

choking hazards, 35
    first, 52
vestibular sense, 43
video, to document child's
    eating, 197
vision impairment, 207–8
visual sense, 37–39
vitamin D, 118
vocabulary, 141–42
    See also language
volume-driven feeding, 15
vomiting, 203, 204

W
waking up hungry at night, 159
Wall Street Journal, 107
washing child's face, 19–20,
    153–54
water
    6 months, 92
    12 to 36 months, 115–16
    24 to 36 months, 172–74
    encouraging toddlers to
        drink, 172–74
    infused, 174
    testing your, 57
watermelon chunks, 36
weaning
    baby-led, 13–14, 18, 73
    bottle, 95, 134–35
    from pacifiers, 94–95, 135–37
websites, 213–14
Weeks, Caroline, 17–18
weight loss, 62
wheat, 58
wigglers (eater type), 98
World Health Organization
    (WHO), 7–8, 70, 120

Y
yogurt, freezing, 123

Z
Zimmels, Stacy, 70–71

About the Author

MELANIE POTOCK, MA, CCC-SLP, is an international speaker on the topic of feeding children, from babies to teens. She has coached over a thousand parents to raise healthy, happy eaters right from the start and has over twenty years of clinical experience helping children with pediatric feeding disorders. Melanie is the coauthor of the award-winning *Raising a Healthy, Happy Eater* and the author of *Adventures in Veggieland* and three other books for both parents and children. Melanie's advice has been shared in a variety of television and print media, including *The New York Times*, *Wall Street Journal*, *Washington Post*, CNN.com, and *Parents* magazine. Melanie lives with her family in Colorado.

mymunchbug.com | ⊙mymunchbug_melaniepotock